Handbook of Sports

Rowing

D1129018

RENEWALS 458-4574
DATE DUE

GAYLORD			PRINTED IN U.S.A.

Handbook of Sports Medicine and Science
Rowing

EDITED BY

Niels H. Secher
and
Stefanos Volianitis

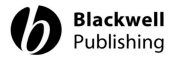

First published 2007

3   2008

Library of Congress Cataloging-in-Publication Data

Rowing / edited by Niels H. Secher and Stefanos Volianitis.
     p. ; cm. — (Handbook of sports medicine and science)
   Includes bibliographical references and index.
   ISBN 978-1-4051-5373-7 (alk. paper)
  1. Rowing–Physiological aspects–Handbooks, manuals, etc.   I. Secher, Niels H.   II. Volianitis, Stefanos S.
III. IOC Medical Commmission. Sub-Commission on Publications in the Sport Sciences.   IV. Series.
   [DNLM: 1. Sports--physiology.   2. Biomechanics.   3. Nutrition.   4. Sports Medicine. QT 260 R882 2007]

   RC122'.R67R69 2007
   797.12'3–dc22

2006037653

ISBN 978-1-4051-5373-7

A catalogue record for this title is available from the British Library

Set in 8.75/12pt Stone Serif by SNP Best-set Typesetter Ltd., Hong Kong
Printed and bound in Malaysia by Vivar Printing Sdn Bhd

Commissioning Editor: Gina Almond
Editorial Assistant: Victoria Pittman
Development Editor: Adam Gilbert
Production Controller: Debbie Wyer

For further information on Blackwell Publishing, visit our website:
http://www.blackwellpublishing.com

Contents

List of Contributors

Zenon B. Babraj MA
University of Southern California, Los Angeles, CA
90089-0602, USA

Richard Budgett MA, MBBS
Olympic Medical Institute, Northwick Park Hospital,
Harrow, Middlesex HA1 3UJ, UK

Louise Burke PhD, APD
Department of Sports Nutrition, Australian Institute of
Sport, Belconnen, ACT 2617, Australia

Sandra L. Dupcak PsyD
Clinical Sport Psychologist, Framingham, MA 01701,
USA

Dries M. Hettinga MSc, PhD
School of Health Sciences and Social Care, Brunel
University, Uxbridge UB8 3PH, UK

Kurt Jensen MSc
Team Danmarks Testcenter, Institute of Sports Science
and Clinical Biomechanics, University of Southern
Denmark, Odense M 5230, Denmark

Jaak Jürimäe PhD
Institute of Sport Pedagogy and Coaching Sciences,
University of Tartu, 51014 Tartu, Estonia

Toivo Jürimäe PhD
Institute of Sport Pedagogy and Coaching Sciences,
University of Tartu, 51014 Tartu, Estonia

Valery Kleshnev PhD
National Biomechanics Lead, English Institute of Sport,
Bisham Abbey National Sports Centre, Bisham,
Buckinghamshire SL7 1RT, UK

Jarek Maestu PhD
Institute of Sport Pedagogy and Coaching Sciences,
University of Tartu, 51014 Tartu, Estonia

Henning Bay Nielsen MD, DMSc
Department of Anesthesia, University of Copenhagen,
Rigshospitalet 20041, Copenhagen, DK-2100, Denmark

Niels H. Secher MD, DMSc
Department of Anesthesia, University of Copenhagen,
Rigshospitalet 2041, Copenhagen, DK-2100, Denmark

Juergen Steinacker MD, PhD
Sektion Sport und Rehabilitionsmedizin, Universität
sklinikum Ulm, 89070 Ulm, Germany

Thomas Vogelsang MSc
Department of Anesthesia, University of Copenhagen,
Rigshospitalet 20041, Copenhagen, DK-2100, Denmark

Stefanos Volianitis PhD
School of Sport and Education, Brunel University,
Uxbridge UB8 3PH, UK

Chie Yoshiga MEd
Department of Anesthesia, University of Copenhagen,
Rigshospitalet 20041, Copenhagen, DK-2100, Denmark

Forewords

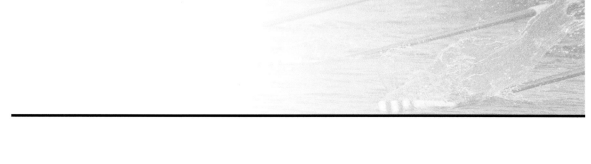

I am pleased to welcome the Handbook on Rowing to the IOC Medical Commission's series, *Handbook of Sports Medicine and Science*.

During the past fifty years, the research literature in sports medicine and the sports sciences has produced a great amount of valuable information about the medical and scientific aspects of rowing. This includes the health and welfare of the athletes as well as the physiology, biomechanics, nutrition, and psychology that are so important to the conditioning programs and actual competition of rowers. The co-editors and the contributing authors have carefully reported on the most up-to-date scientific information that is available and have included practical applications. This valuable information can be utilized by medical doctors, allied health personnel, coaches, sports scientists, as well as rowers of all ages and abilities.

This volume constitutes a major contribution to the literature on sports medicine and the sports sciences. It will serve as the major source of information on the medicine and science of rowing for many years to come. My sincere congratulations go out to all who have been involved in the production of this outstanding publication.

Dr Jacques Rogge
IOC President

As President of FISA, the International Rowing Federation, it is a pleasure to welcome this new publication on the sport of rowing to the IOC Medical Commission's series, *Handbook of Sports Medicine and Science*. FISA was the first Olympic international sports federation, founded in June 1892. Rowing has been a part of the Olympic movement since the first modern Olympic Games and is one of only five sports to have been in every Olympic Games since then.

Rowing also has a strong image as a healthy, all round and clean sport. FISA's Sports Medicine Commission has always been at the forefront of sports medicine and there are numerous former rowers leading the way in medical research and science around the world, including all those who have made this book possible.

I am grateful to all those who have contributed to this outstanding new contribution to sport science.

Denis Oswald
FISA President

Preface

It was the British Nobel laureate A.V. Hill who stated that "some of the most consistent physiological data are contained, not in books on physiology, not even in books on medicine, but in the world's records for running different horizontal distances". Olympic sports require the ultimate from the athlete and, with the engagement of virtually all muscles in the body during rowing, rowing exemplifies the power that humans can achieve. Thus, numerous physiologic variables in integrative human physiology reach their extreme value during "all-out" rowing and some of these data are presented in this text. The ambition of the text has been to provide feed-back to the athletes on the data gathered not only for a scientific purpose but also to guide and help athletes and coaches in their training, testing and team selection. Many, if not all, competitive rowers will have knowledge of their own physiologic profile and it is hoped that the text will help them by providing a perspective on that profile.

The text also provides more general information on the history and organization of rowing and regattas that is considered to help the novice rower and the rower participating in a national, or international, regatta for the first time. Similarly, this text will be useful to the recreational rower, those involved in competitions on the sea, and those continuing rowing throughout life.

The first attempt to present sports-related physiologic data to athletes was by Bengt Saltin and co-workers in Stockholm who around 1970 published a series of reports under the sponsorship of the insurance company Trygg-Hansa. It is an honour that the International Olympic Committee has made it possible to include rowing in the series of Olympic Handbooks. This publication of rowing would not have been possible without the diplomatic efforts of Howard Knuttgen, Boston, USA, a long time friend of Scandinavian exercise physiology. The basis for the text, however, is the oarsmen who have participated in numerous, often complicated and even sophisticated, physiologic experiments. We thank the oarsmen for their enthusiasm and hope that some of them will be inspired by the text to reveal new aspects of the fascinating sport of rowing.

Niels H. Secher
Stefanos Volianitis
2007

Chapter 1
History

S. Volianitis and N.H. Secher

> "When one rows, it's not the rowing which moves the ship: rowing is only a magical ceremony by means of which one compels a demon to move the ship."
>
> Nietzsche

Development of rowing

In parallel with the two milestones in the development of human transportation on land—the domestication of animals and the discovery of the wheel—the construction of water-borne vessels enabled the transport of large amounts of goods long before the development of extensive road networks. The effective use of leverage which facilitates propulsion of even large boats and ships independent of the direction of the wind established the oar as the most cost-effective means of transportation. Even though the first representation of a rowing boat dates to 5800 BC in Finland, larger trading boats propelled by oars were developed by the Phoenicians and the Egyptians in ~3000 BC. Rowing cane boats by means of long oars can be seen in frescoes from the 5th Dynasty of the Pharaohs in Egypt in 2500 BC and an inscription in the tomb of Amenophis II shows him rowing ~1430 BC. Representative cultures where rowing was important, as illustrated in times of war, were the ancient Greeks, the Romans, the Vikings and the Venetians.

Large rowing vessels were used for transport and fighting sea battles in ancient Greece and Rome, but neither the Olympic nor the Spartathlon games included on-water competitions. The earliest record of a rowing race, *The Aeneiad*, written between 30 and 19 BC by Virgil, describes a competition in the Greek fleet that was in Troy around 800 BC. Also, there is evidence that more than 100 boats and 1900 oarsmen participated in rowing regattas organized by the Roman Emperors Augustus and Claudius. A reconstruction of an Athenian *trieres* (three rows of oars; Fig. 1.1), the warship of the classical world, 37 m long and 5.5 m wide with up to 170 oarsmen, named *Olympias*, was built in Piraeus in 1987 and was used in the torch relay of the 2004 Olympic Games in Athens (Fig. 1.2).

Because modern humans are on average approximately 20 cm taller than ancient Greeks, the construction of a craft with the precise dimensions of the ancient vessel led to cramped rowing conditions and, consequently, restrictions on the crew's ability to propel the vessel with full efficiency. Accordingly, the ancient speed records stand unbroken. Without use of the sails and aided by a hull structure similar to the "bulb" of modern large commercial boats her speed reached 8.9 knots. Such speed allowed the *trieres* ("spear ship" according to Aeschylus) to gather momentum to ram enemy ships with her bronze ram fixed on the prow at the water line, and distinguished her from the *pentecontor*, which had 50 oarsmen and two rows of oars. These ships were light for their size and, in contrast to the Roman and North African fleets, the Greek boats were propelled by freemen. Rowing takes its name from the "wineglass" outboard

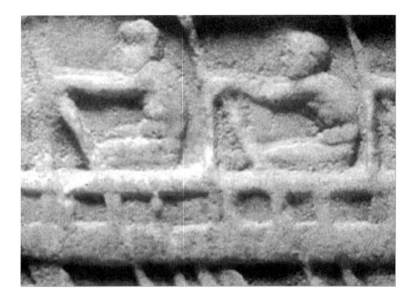

Fig. 1.1 Detail from the Lenormant relief, the most famous pictorial evidence for a three-banked Greek galley, which can be seen in the museum of the Athenian Acropolis.

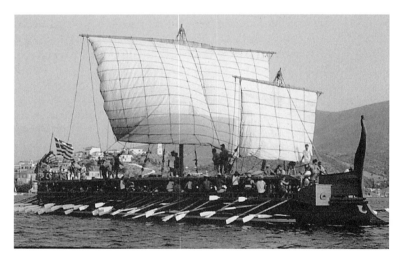

Fig. 1.2 *The Olympias*, a reconstruction of the *trieres*, used for the torch relay of the 2004 Olympic Games.

arrangement of the rows of oars placed one above the other.

Similarly, rowing and sailing were integrated in other parts of the world. The longboat, of which the largest was *Ormen hin Lange* which accommodated 60 rowers, was a major factor in the conquering success of the Vikings (Fig. 1.3). These ships, characterized by planks fastened to a skeleton with wooden or iron nails, were fast and able to handle both the open seas and rivers. Their shallow draft meant that fully loaded boats could be sailed in water only

0.9 m deep and they could be put ashore. The longboats also had intricately carved decorations on the bow; often a dragon, hence, the name *drakkar*, while at the right near side of the ship was a large paddle tied to the hull for steering, giving the term "starboard" from *steor*, rudder or steering paddle, and *bord*, the side of the ship. Records of these ships trace them back to the 8th century AD when the Vikings commuted between North America, Italy and Constantinopole (Istanbul). Rowing competitions on the lakes of Sweden involve *Kyrkbåtar*

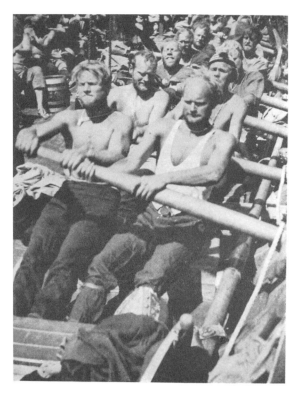

Fig. 1.3 Rowing the *Hugin*, a replica of the Norwegian Gokstad Viking ship on display in Bygdøy, Oslo.

(church boats) which were used to carry parishioners across the lakes, while boats of similar construction were used for fishing along the coast of Norway and the Faroe Islands.

With the (re-)establishment of trade routes between Asia and Europe, Venice became a dominant power in the eastern Mediterranean from ~1200 to ~1500 AD, a status that was secured by the *longship*, a maneuverable warship that used both sail and oars. The Venetians as well as the Romans, Carthaginians and the Knights of Malta all had extensive fleets of rowing galleys, the most famous being the *great galley*, a huge merchant ship with a similar shape to the longship but wider and deeper. While most galleys were rowed *al scaloccio*, meaning that men on a bench pulled on the same oar, the Venetian galley was rowed *alla sensile*, where three men sharing the same bench each had an oar.

The first recorded regatta was organized in Venice in 1315 by the Doge Giovanni Soranzo to celebrate the glory of the Serenissima and the name originates from a festival with *gondolas*. This ~11 m long and ~1.4 m wide boat is rowed by a single standing *gondoliere* who faces the direction of travel while the oar is not fixed into the oarlock, so that it can be withdrawn and used in narrow and crowded canals. The present shape of the gondola, where one side is larger than the other, allowing the vessel to turn on its own axis, was developed in the 1880s by Domenico Tramontin. A popular race in the Grand Canal of Venice is the Vogalonga, which is a 30-km competition for any vessel moved by oars.

Reconstructions of traditional rowing boats are used for sport, pleasure or in ceremonies throughout the world, while original boats are on display in the museums of Paris, Roskilde, Greenwich, Oslo, Dublin and Barcelona.

A long tradition of rowing can also be found in Malta since the Knights of St. John in 1642. The unique feature of Maltese rowing is that two men sit in the bow facing the back and pull while two others stand in the stern and push. Also, traditional "races" took place in the water where "knights" with oared boats replaced the horse. Such matches still take place in France and Denmark (Fig. 1.4).

Another rowing competition in *traineras*, sardine fishing boats manned by 12 rowers and a cox, began in 1879 in San Sebastian, Spain. Since then racing developed into a major betting event and remains popular among more than 35 clubs along the Basque coast. The races, which are rowed in four lanes round a stake, 2.8 km each way, take place in rivers, harbors and at sea. The distinguishing characteristic of these boats is that they are capable of rowing in heavy seas thanks to the *palka* or "false bows," a sock-like breakwater which is fitted over the bow.

Olympic rowing

Race rowing is the oldest modern organized sport and originated in England during the reign of Henry VII (1509–1547) among the Thames professional watermen licensed by the Crown (1555). In 1714, an Irish actor founded the (Thomas) Doggett Coat and Badge boat race for professional bargemen held over 7.4 km on the Thames. The first international fours regatta took place in 1825 between England's Thames watermen and New York rowers in the

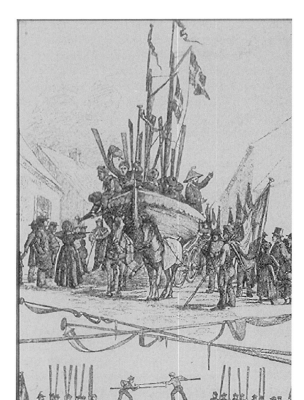

Fig. 1.4 Danish sea contest.

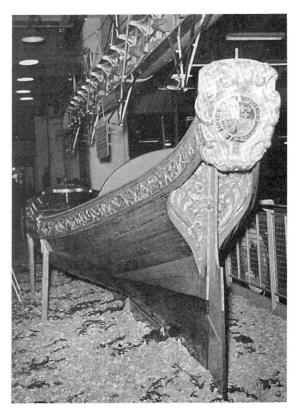

Fig. 1.5 An eight-oared coque. Reproduced from Cleaver, H. (1957) *A History of Rowing.* Herbert Jenkins, London, with permission.

American Star while the first international amateur eights race took place in 1858 between England and France.

In 1778, an eight-oared race took place in London, in boats called "coques," between naval officers returning to college from the Brest blockade fleet during the Napoleonic wars (Fig. 1.5).

The first recorded Procession of the Boats was held in 1793 at Eton College, a boy's school located on the Thames at Windsor, where groups from the same master's house obtained a boat for pleasure or a contest with another house. Oxford University established rowing in 1822, Cambridge in 1827, and the first Boat Race took place in 1829 over 7.75 km on the Thames from Putney to Mortlake.

The Royal Henley Regatta was established in 1839 and has been held annually, except during the two world wars. While it was originally staged as a public attraction revolving around a fair, the emphasis changed so that competitive amateur rowing became the main purpose. The Regatta received royal sponsorship in 1851 and occupies a unique status by maintaining its own rules rather than being under the jurisdiction of the English Rowing Federation or the Fédération Internationale des Sociétés d'Aviron (FISA). Henley operates a heat system with only two boats racing, which entails the organization of up to 100 races on 5 days. The length of the course is 2112 m (Fig. 1.6).

The Head of the River race, funded by Steve Fairbairn (Fig. 1.7) in 1926, also takes place on the Thames on the same course and distance as the Boat Race but in the opposite direction (i.e., from Mortlake to Putney). It is the largest rowing event for eights, with the entries limited to 420. On the

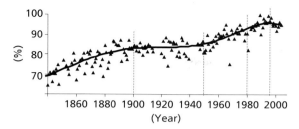

Fig. 1.6 Rowing speed (percent of fastest) from the records of the Grand Challenge Cup (M8+) of the Royal Henley Regatta.

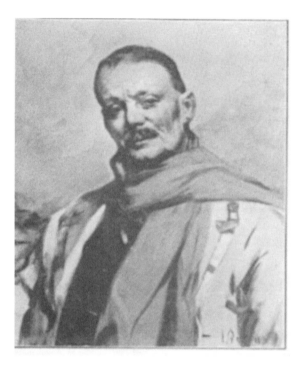

Fig. 1.7 Steve Fairbairn.

same course similar events with comparable participation are organized for singles, pairs and fours also for women and veteran rowers.

Another type of race is the *bumps*, as held in Oxford and Cambridge for example, where all the crews are lined up along the river at set intervals, and start at the same time aiming to catch up with the boat in front and gain a *bump*. Then both crews pull to the side, as they take no further part in that race. In the following race, the bumping crew starts ahead of the crew that was bumped. The *bumps* are held over several days and the position at the end of the last race determines the position on the first day of the race the following year. Also, there are *Town Bumps* races in both cities, open to all crews.

USA

The first organized boat races in the USA took place in New York in the mid 1700s by professional bargemen. Amateur clubs were formed in Boston, New York and Philadelphia in the 1830s. The University of Pennsylvania (The College, Academy and Educational Trust) rowing history dates to 1760, when a challenge was issued to New York to a 6-mile race. The Amateur Boatclub held a regatta on the Schuylkill on November 12, 1835, in which the Blue Devil club rowed a boat of that name, and seven eight-oared barges took part.

However, the dominant organization of rowing in the USA came from universities when Harvard and Yale started rowing in 1843 and 1844, respectively, and first raced each other in eight-oared shells in 1852 over a distance of 7.4 km. The Head of the Charles in Boston is the world's largest rowing event and was initiated on October 16, 1965. Today more than 5400 athletes from around the world compete in 19 events over a distance of 5.6 km.

Germany

Rowing came to Germany through Hamburg (1836) following an initiative of British rowers. The German Rowing Association (Deutscher Ruderverband, DRV) was established in March 1883 and lightweight rowing races were introduced in Germany in 1925. After World War II there were two German rowing teams and rowing associations, DRV and DRSV (1965–1991), but with the fall of the Berlin wall in November 1989 they were reunited in 1991.

Rowing in northern Europe and Scandinavia is not only about competing in racing shells, but is also a leisure sport practiced in inriggers where oarlocks are on the side of the boat (Fig. 1.8).

Many clubs developed an interest in the leisure rowing scene, *wanderrudern*, with trips being organized on splendid waterways. Long distance tours

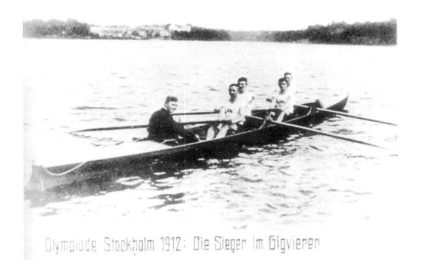

Olympiade Stockholm 1912: Die Sieger im Gigvierer

Fig. 1.8 The Danish inrigger four winning the 1912 Olympic regatta in Stockholm. Reproduced from Meuret, J.-L. (1992) *The FISA Centenary Book*. Fédération Internationale des Sociétés d'Aviron, Oberhofen am Thunersee.

and gig races were also introduced to the regatta schedules. National and club championships in two- and four-oared inriggers encompass races from 500 m to 50 km.

Italy

A significant Italian contribution to the development of race rowing was the buoy system for courses, named Albano after the city in the northwest of Italy. The system encompasses a series of small buoys on the side of each racing lane, which are 15 m apart and run the length of the course. The buoys start out red for 100 m, turn to white and then back to red for the final 100 m, with one red buoy for each 500 m. On a six-lane 2000 m course, this is accomplished by a grid of wires about 1.2 m below the surface of the water suspended by the small buoys and a few larger ones. These cables are anchored on each end, pulled with 100 kg and stabilized by lateral cables and anchors at each 500 m junction, resulting in a symmetrical formation referred to as "military cemetery," meaning that the buoys are aligned both across and diagonally.

Holland

The first manmade rowing course, built at Bosbaan, Amsterdam, in 1936 for the Olympic Games, originally had five lanes but was widened to six even

bigger lanes in 1954 for the European Championships, which was the first international event where races for women were included, and today it features eight lanes. The first "European Championships" for single sculls (the Holland Becker) was introduced on August 14, 1886 and takes place annually as part of a regatta with that name (Fig. 1.9).

Australia

The first rowing race in Australia took place on May 16, 1818, when a four-oared gig stroked by John Piper won a race from Bradley's Head on the north shore of Sydney Harbour, to Sydney Cove. The Melbourne University Boat Club was established in 1859. The first official race for eights took place on March 6, 1878, on the lower Yarra, where a crew from the Mercantile Club in Sydney, representing New South Wales, was defeated by a crew from the Victorian Rowing Association. The Australian Henley with a series of Challenge Cups has been run by the Melbourne Amateur Regatta Association annually since 1904, except during the two world wars. In its heyday, the Australian Henley ranked with the Melbourne Cup and Australian Football League grand final as a major sporting event including an inter-university contest for a cup presented by Oxford and Cambridge oarsmen and a social occasion where a Miss Henley contest was held.

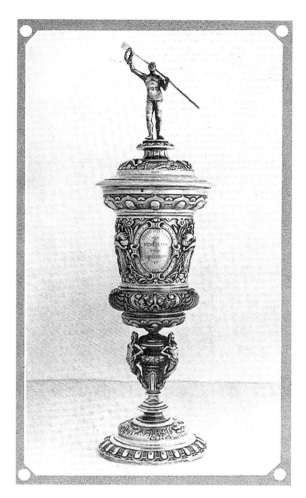

Fig. 1.9 The Holland Becker.

Japan

Rowing came early to the Far East with the first rowing club in 1866 and the first rowing regatta in Kobe on December 24, 1870.

Rowers and achievements

As the cultural and sociologic status of sport in general is changing, the increased commercialization of all Olympic sports in the last 20 years has enabled rowers to compete for longer. While Jack Beresford's career span and achievement — five medals in successive Olympic Games from 1920 to 1936 — was unprecedented for his time, today several international rowers have succeeded in com-

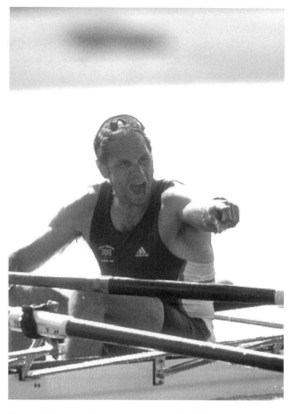

Fig. 1.10 Steven Redgrave winning his fifth gold medal at the 2000 Olympic Games.

bining a professional and a rowing career, with the average age of Olympic rowers in the late twenties. At the Sydney Olympics, Steven Redgrave at the age of 38 won a fifth successive gold medal (Fig. 1.10). Similarly, James Tomkins of Australia, the only rower to win World Championship titles in every sweep oar event, and Elisabeta Lipa of Romania, who holds the rowing record for most Olympic medals won (eight, five of them gold), were both at end of their thirties (Fig. 1.11).

Coastal and ocean rowing

Coastal and ocean rowing is a type of rowing performed on the sea. Because of the harsher conditions encountered at sea, the boats are wider and more robust than those used on rivers and lakes. Coastal rowing was developed out of sea-going versions of racing shells, the *gigs*. These four-oared vessels were not only light enough to be launched from a ship's deck by two men, but they were also fast and suitable for carrying pilots to ships in rough weather. Professional gig racing began in the 1840s and thrived until the 20th century. These pilot boats were the forefathers of the revival of pleasure and competition sea rowing in New York, San Francisco, Finland and Sweden.

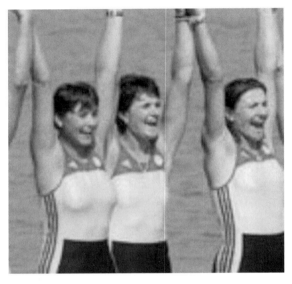

Fig. 1.11 Elisabeta Lipa (center), the most decorated rower.

Within the Guinness Book of Records' ideology of first and fastest, sea rowing events are created, for example from the Faro Islands to Copenhagen rowed by Joensen in 1987 (3093 km in 41 days). The Atlantic Ocean was first successfully rowed by the Norwegians George Harboe and Gabriel Samuelsen in 1896 and since then it has become an organized challenge for singles, doubles and fours, with the present record for the single being 42 days and 13 hours by the Frenchman Emmanuel Coindre using an east to west route (www.oceanrowing.com).

In the Netherlands, *sloeproeien*, rowing in lifeboats and Navy instruction longboats, is well developed, thus allowing for the preservation and restoration of traditional boats. As all boats are different, there is a system for time correction with a C-value to obtain comparable results.

The sport of coastal and offshore rowing is thriving across Europe, although at present most British sea rowing is "traditional" fixed seat rowing and competition is of a regional nature (Fig. 1.12). France is leading the development of modern sliding seat sea boats, *yoles*, and national competition is well established. With the establishment of the FISA World Rowing Coastal Challenge, the use of the French *yole* is gaining popularity and most European countries have adopted this type of boat. The event is open to club rowers without pre-

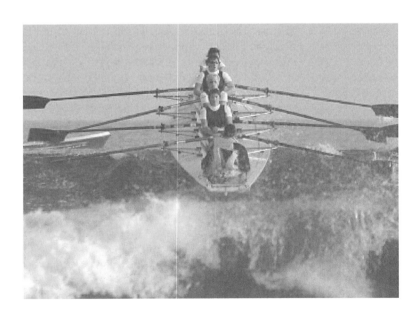

Fig. 1.12 A coxed four *yole* riding on high surf.

qualification, in this way acknowledging the participatory nature of coastal rowing and confirming FISA's support of sea rowing traditions through rough water competitions that require seamanship and navigation in addition to technical skills. Boat categories include the single, the double and the coxed four.

This competition is considerably different from Olympic rowing. No lanes are defined and the course is triangular with a total distance of 6000 m. Women cover the course once and men twice, with only one race per boat category. The first FISA Coastal Rowing World Championship event is planned for 2007.

In North America, the sport of "open water" rowing relies on longer, lighter and faster boats while having an emphasis on safety through the use of positive flotation and self-bailing capacity, supplemented by the rower's seamanship skills. North American boats do not conform to the minimum standards established by FISA because they are too long and do not weigh enough. Open water racing in North America is popular in New England, California and Washington. The pre-eminent open water race in New England is the Blackburn Challenge.

The Cornish Pilot Gig Association (CPGA) is the largest British sea rowing group and preserves a tradition using both original and new boats made to a closely controlled specification. The CPGA has seen a continuing growth over the past decade or so and new boats are constantly being built. The Cornish gig has been adopted by rowers in the Netherlands and there is a successful gig club in Wales.

The 22-mile London Great River Race is the major British event for traditional boats attracting up to 350 crews, but there are many regular events throughout the long March to October season. The Welsh Longboat Rowing Association, for instance, organizes a total of 21 offshore and estuary events each year. These range from 5-mile league races to the Celtic Challenge rowing race, an epic Irish Sea crossing. The Celtic Challenge rowing race is a gruelling 90-mile rowing race from Arklow in Ireland to Aberystwyth in Wales. It is classed as the longest sea rowing race in the world. It is a biannual event, which usually takes place on the first Saturday in May with crews from Wales, Ireland, England and as far afield as Germany.

Celtic sea rowers in Wales and Ireland have adopted modern designs of fixed seat boats, loosely based on the Irish *curragh*, which is still used by sea rowers in both countries. The annual All-Ireland Coastal Rowing Championships involves up to 350 crews each year and is believed to be second in size only to the CPGA in the Scilly Isles. The New Celtic Design boat which was introduced only 4 years ago is gaining in popularity and is used as a bridge to link the various Irish classes of boats. However, since 2006 FISA dimensions are followed in hull design.

Surf boat rowing is popular in Australia and New Zealand and to a lesser extent South Africa. Usually associated with surf life-saving clubs, surf boat crews are trained in life-saving skills as well as learning to be competent oarsman. The Australian form of the sport attracts wide media coverage and is often featured on mainstream sporting shows in the summer months. Surf boats are four-oared vessels with a pointed bow and stern. The boat is steered by a sweep who stands in the bow and uses an oar-like rudder to control the boat (Fig. 1.13).

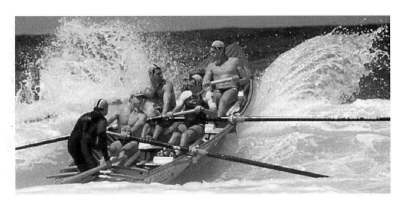

Fig. 1.13 The start of a surf boat competition at Bondi Beach, Australia.

Table 1.1 Age categories for Masters rowing.

A	27–35 (31–35 in the UK)
B	36–42
C	43–49
D	50–54
E	55–59
F	60–64
G	65–69
H	70–74

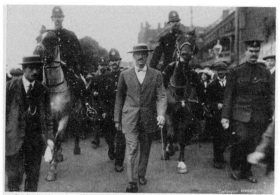

In the heyday of professional sculling, Ernest Barry's arrival on the towpath at Putney necessitated this kind of escort. The year—1913. The occasion—after Barry's race with H. Pearce of Australia for £500 aside, which Barry won.

During competition, surf crews start on the beach and row through the surf, proceed to a certain number of turning points (referred to as the can) and then race back to the beach. As the boat nears the beach oars are raised and the boat is literally surfed ashore. Surf boat races are conducted on a weekly basis throughout the Australian summer with hundreds of crews participating.

Masters rowing

Masters (or veteran in the UK) rowers classifications begin at 27 years of age and the distance covered is 1000 m. Masters events also include a letter designation indicating the average age of the crew in years (Table 1.1).

Professional rowing

The first English professional sculling championship race was held in London in 1831 between two watermen, C. Campbell and J. Williams. From 1831 to 1952 there has been a World Professional Championship, with R. Arnst from New Zealand and E. Barry from England (Fig. 1.14) dominating in the early 19th century. Arnst beat Barry in a 3.25-mile race above the Victoria Falls on the Zambezi River in 1910 in what may have been the first serious high altitude competition. During the 1870s and 1880s, professional sculling was a major attraction on Lake Victoria, Canada, where the first organized club with some 75 members was founded in 1865. Early records of rowing in Whitehall boats include reference to an 1859 race on the Gorge Waterway and Inner Harbor.

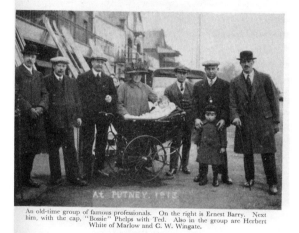

An old-time group of famous professionals. On the right is Ernest Barry. Next him, with the cap, "Bossie" Phelps with Ted. Also in the group are Herbert White of Marlow and C. W. Wingate.

Fig. 1.14 Ernest Barry after racing H. Pearce of Australia in 1913 for £500 at Putney.

Development of equipment

Boat design and materials

Early racing boats were descended from the clinker built boats of the English river Thames, and the New York Whitehall skiffs, named after Whitehall St. at the Battery. These boats were often involved in betting races. Henry Clasper of Oxford built the first keel-less boats and spoon-shaped oars in 1848. Some early Schuylkill boats had staggered rowing seats with wicker ladies seats alongside the rowers. Up to this time the largest sweep racing shell were six-men boats without a coxswain although there were 10 and 12 person shells built in England. The last six-oared barge race recorded in Philadelphia was in 1884. Wood boats were the norm, although pressed paper boats were made in the 1870s and aluminum boats in the 1920s. George Pocock, the son of the Eton School boatbuilder, immigrated to Seattle and produced wood shells from 1920 to 1960, and became known as the father of American rowing. Compost carbon fiber, Kevlar® and epoxy resins boats developed rapidly in the 1970s, and minimum weight requirements were introduced by FISA to control the cost of the lightweight shells (Table 1.2).

Around 1828 Anthony Brown in England developed riggers, used at bow and stern, to compensate for the narrowing of the boats and to increase leverage. Boat speed is significantly improved with the use of sliding riggers, where the body mass remains fixed while the rigger or foot-stretcher unit slides. When the body mass is stationary, the boat does not pitch bow to stern as much, thus less hull resistance is created and rowing efficiency is increased. The sliding rigger concept dates back to 1877 when Michael Davis of Portland, Maine, USA, used a

sliding footboard and outriggers with a fixed seat to eliminate the excessive friction from the loaded (body weighted) moving seat. The sliding rigger concept was tried in the 1920s by Walter Hoover (USA), and in 1954 by C.E. Poynter of Bedford (UK). *The Illustrated London News* of September 25, 1954, described the invention of a double scull. The concept surfaced again in 1960 when Nick Smith (Australia) fitted a practice boat with a sliding rigger system and the FISA single championship in 1981 was won in a boat with a sliding rigger by Michael Kolbe (Fig. 1.15). However, that construction was

Table 1.2 Classes of boat recognized by the Fédération Internationale des Sociétés d'Aviron (FISA) and their minimum weight in kilograms.

Single Sculls (1×)	14
Double Sculls (2×)	27
Pair (2−)	27
Coxed Pair (2+)	32
Quadruple Sculls (4×)	52
Four (4−)	50
Coxed Four (4+)	51
Eight (8+)	96

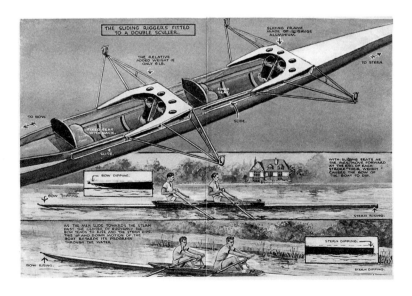

Fig. 1.15 Sliding rigger.

banned by FISA in 1983 because it was thought to be more costly than sliding seat boats.

Mitchel Davis of Yale invented the swivel oarlock. The slide with wheels has been variously attributed to Dr. Schiller of Berlin (1863), the Canadian Ed Hanlin and Captain John Babcock and was first used in a crew boat in 1870. Walter Brown of England raced a sliding seat single in 1861. Before that time the same effect was accomplished by sluicing the seat with grease and sliding on leather bottom trousers.

From around 1965, some crews preferred to have the coxswain positioned lying down in the front of the boat rather than sitting at the end of the boat. By doing so the cox's body becomes more stable with the variation in the speed of the boat through each stroke and the view of the course is obviously enhanced. On the other hand, the cox has less control of the crew and the arrangement is therefore more popular for pairs and fours than eights, although this limitation is compensated for with the introduction of microphones rather than a megaphone for inboard communication.

Blade design

The early oars were straight with a very long flattened surface and square looms but in the 1700s oars became a little more contoured with a curve to the blade, but still a long slender blade. In the 1800s and the 1900s many blade shapes, "Macon" being the most popular, were used to make oars with different materials: wood, aluminum and composite materials (fiberglass, carbon fiber, Kevlar). The challenge using composite materials in the 1970s was to make an oar that would perform, be durable and be cost effective. In 1972, a British company, Guest, Keen and Nettlefolds, produced a set of carbon reinforced oars; however, they were very costly. In 1977, the Dreissigacker brothers, Dick and Pete manufactured carbon fiber oars and later developed a composite oar that became the choice of all North America and much of the rest of the world market. In the fall of 1991 the Dreissigackers introduced the asymmetrical *hatchet blade* (Fig. 1.16) design that took its name from its cleaver-like shape. Today, many manufacturers are producing the hatchet blade ("big blade") that has become the standard in racing rowing.

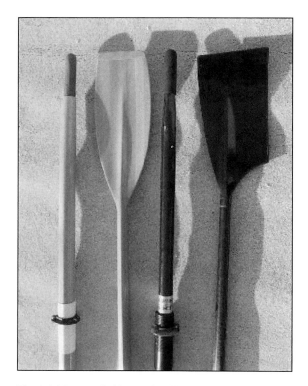

Fig. 1.16 Macon (left) and "big blade" (right) oars.

Rowing ergometers

Rowing machines have been in use since the mid 19th century as evidenced by a patent for a rowing machine by William Curtis in 1871. Ergometers have been used in rowing training since the 1950s and 1960s in many countries

The introduction of the Gamut ergometer to the USA initiated changes in training and selection processes. The 1980s saw the development of some lighter ones, such as the Repco, which had a wheel that acted against air resistance. Some years later, the Norwegian Gjessing ergometer became the accepted standard measuring device around the world. In 1980, a rowing ergometer using a bicycle wheel, a wooden handle and an odometer was developed in the USA as an off-water rowing training aid. This ergometer was used by CRASH-B (a group of 1976–1980 US Olympic and World Team athletes) which formed a regatta of about 20 rowers in Harvard's Newell Boathouse (Fig. 1.17).

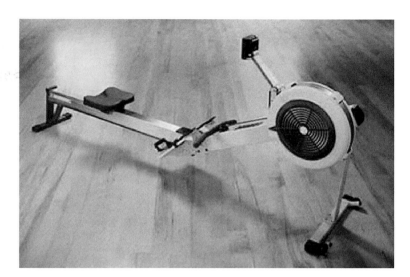

Fig. 1.17 The "Concept II" rowing ergometer.

Today, ergometer competitions have official FISA status with an annual world indoor championship regatta and regional qualifying satellite regattas around the world (Table 1.3).

Most recently, an application of functional electric stimulation (FES) modified on a rowing ergometer has enabled paraplegics to compete in whole body ergometer rowing events. Also, the rowing ergometer has been put on slides to better simulate on-water rowing and the ergometers can then be combined to simulate the teamwork of the pair, four- or eight-oared boat. The work output produced is projected onto a screen, allowing comparisons with other competitors, or can be transmitted via the Internet to facilitate worldwide competitions.

Prior to the widespread use of the rowing ergometer, off-season rowing training was facilitated in rowing tanks encompassing up to eight rowers (Fig. 1.18), although winter training often included "general" cross-training for a balanced body development.

Rowing style

By the turn of the century, rowing style had become a center of controversy. The traditional English orthodox style featured a long straight-backed body swing where, as the crew is pulling together and recovering uniformly, the shell moves faster and further between strokes than it does while the oars

are in the water; thus, control of the recovery enhances the chance of winning (Fig. 1.19).

George Pocock's adage was that "oarsmen must row with the boat," meaning they must not "row faster than the boat is going" otherwise they will rush their slides to attain a higher stroke rate and therefore check at the catch and reduce the run of the boat.

In the USA, Hiram Conibear, an athletic trainer, took over the rowing program at the University of Washington and developed the American Conibear style. This style required a hard quick catch, with shoulders and body vertical within 5–7.6 cm after the catch, a quick zip out of the bow with the arms at the finish, fast first part of the slide slowing at the last moment of the recovery. Conibear, together with George and Dick Pocock, influenced many prominent US coaches of the 20th century.

In England, Steve Fairbairn (1862–1938), a rower in the 1880s and later a coach in the early decades of the 20th century at Jesus College, Cambridge (Fig. 1.7), revolutionized the style of rowing and his coaching had an immense influence on the sport not only in Great Britain. Fairbairn's first principle was that the legs were the strongest part of the body and thus the beginning of the stroke must be characterized by a good leg drive. The oarsman must not think too much about his body but concentrate on correct blade movements and during the recovery the blade must be kept well clear of the water.

Table 1.3 World records for 2000 m ergometer rowing in 2006. Heavyweight (HWT) and lightweight (LWT, 75 kg for men and 61.5 kg for women) status is indicated. Updated records can be found at www.concept2.com.

Age (years)	Weight	Gender	Name	Country	Time
12 & under	Any weight	M	Marian Uroic	Croatia	7:13.2
	HWT	W	Fie Udby	Denmark	7:30.3
	LWT	W	Charlotte Manning	Canada	8:23.1
13–18	HWT	M	Karsten Brodowsky	Germany	5:47.0
		W	Sarah Hubbard	Australia	6:33.9
	LWT	M	Henrik Stephansen	Denmark	6:12.1
		W	Johanne Thomsen	Denmark	7:07.0
19–29	HWT	M	Rob Waddell	New Zealand	5:38.3
		W	Sophie Balmary	France	6:28.4
	LWT	M	Elia Luini	Italy	6:02.6
		W	Jo Hammond	UK	6:57.0
30–39	HWT	M	Matthias Siejkowski	Germany	5:37.0
		W	Sarah Winckless	UK	6:28.8
	LWT	M	Eskild Ebbessen	Denmark	6:06.4
		W	Lisa Schlenker	USA	6:56.7
40–49	HWT	M	Jens Doberschütz	Germany	5:58.4
		W	Carol Skricki	USA	6:48.2
	LWT	M	Mike Caviston	USA	6:18.2
		W	Lisa Schlenker	USA	7:09.6
50–54	HWT	M	Andy Ripley	UK	6:07.7
		W	Anna Bailey	UK	7:06.6
	LWT	M	Graham Watt	New Zealand	6:25.8
		W	Joan Van Blom	USA	7:22.6
55–59	HWT	M	Andy Ripley	UK	6:21.3
		W	Anna Bailey	UK	7:30.0
	LWT	M	Dennis Hastings	USA	6:40.8
		W	Helen Mandley	USA	7:57.2

(*Continued.*)

Table 1.3 *Continued.*

Age (years)	Weight	Gender	Name	Country	Time
60–64	HWT	M	Paul Hendershott	USA	6:23.7
		W	Mies Bernelot Moens	Netherlands	7:33.1
	LWT	M	Roger Prowse	UK	6:48.8
		W	Ingrid Petersen	Denmark	7:48.6
65–69	HWT	M	Peter Lekisch	USA	6:53.2
		W	Renee Camu	France	8:09.8
	LWT	M	Lyle Parker	Australia	6:37.7
		W	Luanne Mills	USA	8:00.0
70–74	HWT	M	Stephen Rounds	USA	7:02.6
		W	Ruth Doell	USA	8:42.2
	LWT	M	Geoffrey Knight	UK	7:13.4
		W	Sarah Keel	USA	8:52.9
75–79	HWT	M	Stephen Rounds	USA	7:22.3
		W	Ruth Doell	USA	8:54.0
	LWT	M	Dean Smith	USA	7:25.3
		W	Mavis Surridge	UK	9:13.1
80–84	HWT	M	Joe Clinard	USA	8:03.5
		W	Gertrude Lowther	USA	10:12.9
	LWT	M	Dean Smith	USA	7:52.5
		W	Jessie Welsh	UK	10:05.5
85–89	HWT	M	Stephen Richardson	USA	9:17.5
	LWT	M	John Hodgson	UK	9:22.0
		W	Jessie Welsh	UK	10:25.2
90–94	HWT	M	George Braceland	USA	11:01.9
	LWT	M	John Hodgson	UK	9:25.8
		W	Ernestine Bayer	USA	12:07.5
95–99	LWT	M	John Hodgson	USA	10:28.1

Fairbairn was the first to train his crews to slide in their seats to maximize the length of their stroke, and his adage that mileage wins races was a precursor of year round on-water training. "The

Fairbairns," a rowing competition for novice rowers held on the River Cam late every autumn, is named after him.

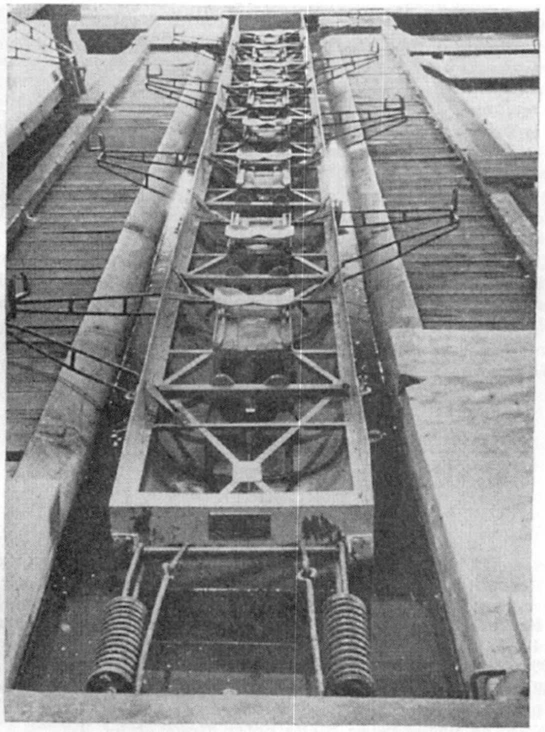

Karl Adam (1912–1976), a professor of rowing and a coach, had a major impact on one of the most successful eras in German rowing history which started at the end of the 1950s (Fig. 1.20). He was co-founder of the Ratzeburger Rowing Club in 1953 and head of the rowing academy there. He was a great innovator of rowing and training techniques and introduced methods that had a major impact on the further development of rowing — known in the rowing world as the "Ratzeburger" style. In the 1960s, Karl Adam's world champion crews from Ratzeburg pioneered advances such as speed play, interval training, shovel-shaped oars and "bucket" rigging (which put the number 4 and 5 oars on the starboard side of the boat; numbers 2 and 3 in the four, respectively). He also introduced longer tracks for the seat to travel forward more than 10 cm past the pin and allow maximal compression of the legs at the catch. Another novelty of Adam was the concept of systematic crew selection from rowers across Germany and his boats won in 1959–67 not less than seven titles at World and European Championships. In addition, his eight won an Olympic gold medal in 1960 in Rome and 1968 in Mexico — introducing the title of "Deutschlandachter." Nothing since has matched the impact of the sudden explosion of Ratzeburg and Karl Adam onto the rowing scene.

Fig. 1.18 An eight-seat rowing tank.

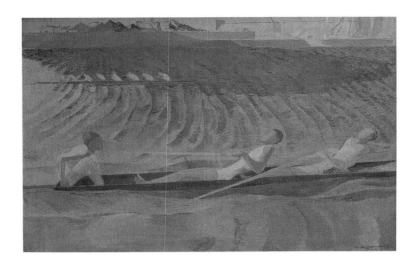

Fig. 1.19 Old time rowing (Harald Hansen, Danish artist).

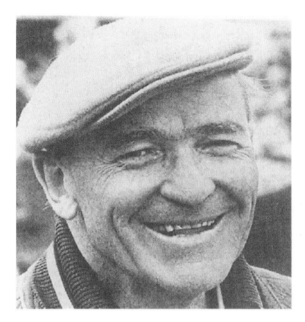

Fig. 1.20 Karl Adam.

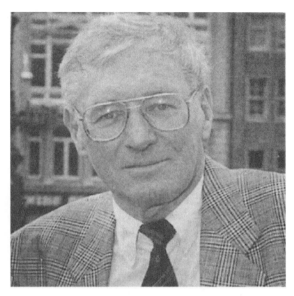

Fig. 1.21 Thor Nilsen.

A significant contribution to the sport of rowing has been made by the world-renowned Norwegian coach Thor Nilsen (Fig. 1.21). Currently FISA's development director, Nilsen is also honorary chairman of the Competitive Rowing Commission and has served both on FISA's Council and Executive Committee. Nilsen has developed national training centres in several countries and has also served as national rowing coach in Norway and Sweden as well as technical director and head coach for Greece, Ireland, Spain and Italy. He has influenced many coaches worldwide and his coaching results include over 40 World Championships and eight Olympic gold medals.

Organization and FISA

History of FISA

FISA was founded in Turin on June 25, 1892, by delegates from France, Belgium, Switzerland, Italy and the Adriatic Federation (alias Austria–Hungary) as the first international amateur team sport governing body and is based in Lausanne, Switzerland.

Early organization of rowing as a sport probably reflects the complexity of storing a large number of boats and therefore the creation of large boathouses establishing a unique club culture (Fig. 1.22).

In 1893, FISA held its first European rowing championship, in Orta, Italy, and then annually until it was replaced by the World Championships (Lucerne, Switzerland, 1962). Similar World Championships regattas were held for Juniors (Ratzeburg, Germany, 1967) and under 23 years (Nations Cup), the latter receiving official FISA status by 2005. By 2006, FISA included 118 national rowing associations. There has also been a one-off North American Championship (1967) while regional continental regattas are held in Latin America, Asia and Africa as part of FISA's development program.

Olympic Games

Because Baron de Coubertin was a keen sculler (Fig. 1.23), rowing was included in the program of the first modern Olympics in 1896 (Athens) but all five events scheduled were cancelled because of bad weather. However, the rowing events did take place in 1900 (Paris) and rowing is one of the five sports to have been in every modern Olympics. In 1912, inrigger fours were in the Olympic program and the

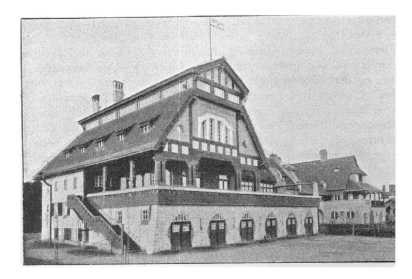

Fig. 1.22 The boathouse at Grunau, Berlin, Germany.

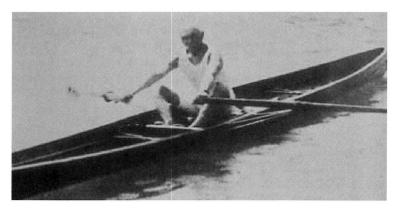

Fig. 1.23 Baron Pierre de Coubertin sculling on Lac Leman.

event was won by Denmark (Fig. 1.8). Women's rowing was added only in 1976 and lightweight events joined the program in 1996. Thus, rowing has managed to maintain the third largest quota after athletics and swimming, having 14 sets of medals and more than 550 participants. In 2005, adaptive rowing was included in the Paralympics, which is also evidence of the growing popularity of the sport.

European Championships

In the 1893 European Rowing Championships there were only three events (men's single, coxed four and eight) and only 10 entries. Races were 3000 m long, except for singles which were only 2000 m.

The last European Rowing Championships took place in 1973 and were open to all countries. In 2006, FISA re-established the European Rowing Championships to start in 2007 at the end of September, and it will feature the 14 Olympic boat classes racing over 2000 m. While the World Championships are maintained as the main FISA annual regatta, the European Championships will be open only to National Rowing Federations from Europe.

Boat types and categories of rowers

From 1896 up to the 1972 Olympic Games rowing included seven male events in the Olympic program

Table 1.4 Rowing events in Olympic Games (OG) and World Championships (WC) programs.

Boat type	Men		Women	
	Heavyweight	**Lightweight**	**Heavyweight**	**Lightweight**
Single scull (1×)	OG	WC	OG	WC
Double scull (2×)	OG	OG	OG	OG
Quad scull (4×)	OG	WC	OG	WC
Pair (2–)	OG	WC	OG	
Four (4–)	OG	OG	WC	
Eight (8+)	OG	WC	OG	
Pair with coxswain (2+)	WC			
Four with coxswain (4+)	WC			

(1×, 2×, 2-, 2+, 4-, 4+, 8+). The 2000 m standard distance was originally defined as the entire length of the racing lane but now is defined as the length between the boat's bowball and the finish line. In 1976 the number of events was increased to 14 as one male event (4×) and six female events (1×, 2×, 4×, 2-, 4-, 8+ over 1000 m distance) were introduced. Women's events were changed to the standard distance of 2000 m in 1984, which made female rowing more aerobic with less demand for strength and power. The current Olympic program was introduced after the 1992 Games, when lightweight events were included (LM2×, LM4-, LW2×) at the expense of M2+, M4+ and W4. Yet, these events are maintained in the World Championships program (Table 1.4). For lightweight men's crews the limit is 70 kg with no rower over 72.5 kg, while for women's crews the limits are 57 and 59 kg, respectively. For single sculls the limits are 72.5 and 59 kg, for men and women, respectively.

The coxswain (or simply the cox) sits in the stern (except in bowloaders) facing the bow, steers the boat and coordinates the power and rhythm of the rowers. As coxswains are members of the crew, a women's crew may not be steered by a man nor may a men's crew be steered by a woman except in masters races. The minimum weight for a coxswain is 55 kg for men's and 50 kg for women's crews. To make up this weight, a coxswain may carry a maximum of 10 kg deadweight, which shall be placed in the boat as close as possible to the coxswain's person.

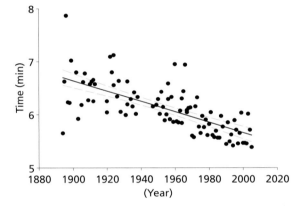

Fig. 1.24 Rowing speed based on Olympic and World Championship records (M8+). Regression line shown.

Trends of rowing performance

Long-term performance in rowing is difficult to analyze, because results are significantly affected by weather conditions and differences between the race courses used in European, World and Olympic events. Yet it is clear that there has been a steady increase in rowing speed over the years, with an average improvement of 0.7 s per year (Table 1.5; Fig. 1.24).

A more detailed presentation of the progress may be obtained by comparison of records from a single regatta, and for that purpose the Royal Henley

Table 1.5 Predicted times for 2007 based on regression lines established from Olympic and World Championship records.

Boat type	Slope of regression	2007 Time
M4+	−0.84	6:07
M2×	−0.75	6:17
M2−	−1.06	6:23
M1×	−0.81	6:46
M2+	−0.93	6:51
M4−	−0.79	5:53
M4×	−0.43	5:47
M8+	−0.60	5:34
ML1×	−0.92	6:54
ML4−	−1.20	5:54
ML8+	−0.78	5:36
W2×	−1.42	6:43
W1×	−1.97	7:10
W4×	−0.31	6:23
W8+	−0.52	6:10
WL1×	−1.22	7:37
WL2×	−1.98	6:55
WL4×	−3.15	6:21
LM4×	−0.57	5:55
LM2×	−2.47	6:07
W4−	−1.30	6:30
W2−	−2.22	6:49
Average	−1.17	6:24

M, men; L, lightweight; W, women; +, with coxswain; −, without coxswain.

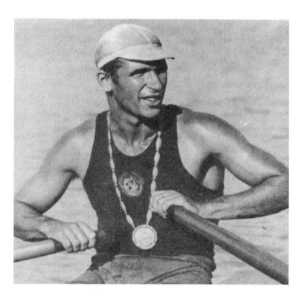

Fig. 1.25 Ivanov, winner of three single scull Olympic championships (1956–1964).

Regatta is ideal because it is the oldest still existing institution in race rowing. From these records it is possible to define the following periods of rowing development, as illustrated in Fig. 1.6.

Before 1900 there was a fast growth in performance of 1–1.5% per year, which may be explained by initial development of equipment (timber boats, outriggers and the sliding seat), in addition to sporting technique and training methods. The slower growth of ~0.5% per year from 1900 to 1950 may have been caused by the two world wars and the amateur status of the athletes. From 1950 to 1980, however, performance grew at a pace of ~1–2% per year. It may be consid-ered that the competition level rose substantially when Eastern block countries joined Olympic sports in 1952. Thus, sport acquired a political dimension with the USSR (Fig. 1.25) followed by the DDR dominating international rowing (as many other sports) for decades.

Only as western societies became richer, a similar (semi-) professional status became widespread and boomed the training volume and methods, while one can only speculate whether the use of drugs in sport has played a part. This performance growth was even faster for women, because it coincided with the introduction of these events (1953).

In the period 1980–96 there was a slower growth of ~0.5–0.8% per year. This growth rate could be reflective of the training volume approaching its biologic limit and an improvement in drug control. However, rowing performance continues to grow relatively faster than in athletics or swimming, possibly because of significant developments in equipment which replaced wooden boats and oars with plastic or carbon fiber and the introduction of the "big blade." Also, the proactive position of FISA on the wider promotion of rowing and the popularization of modern training technologies may have played a part.

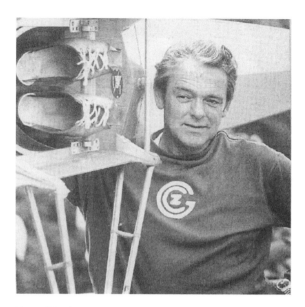

Fig. 1.26 Thomas Keller.

decade has contributed to make the rower much bigger than was the case when international rowing competitions were introduced. As illustrated by the better results for heavy (~93 kg for men) than for lightweight (70 kg) rowing, increasing body size promotes results and, accordingly, selection of national teams among all rowers within the country rather than only within a particular boat club has contributed to make the competitive heavy rower taller and heavier. An effort to standardize the courses used not only for FISA championships but also for local regattas was made largely on the initiative of FISA president Thomas Keller (1962–1976; Fig. 1.26).

Since 1996 results seem to be stable. We can only speculate that further performance development has been limited by strict doping control methods (such as the blood doping test) and, most likely, by the marginal development of rowing material in recent years.

For more than 100 years, it is likely that the increasing size of the population by about 1 cm per

Recommended reading

Cleaver, H. (1957) *A History of Rowing*. Herbert Jenkins, London.

Dodd, C. (1983) *The Oxford Cambridge Boat Race*. Stanley Paul, London.

Dodd, C. (1992) *The Story of World Rowing*. Stanley Paul, London.

Herrick, R.F. (1948) *Red Top, Reminiscences of Harvard Rowing*. Harvard University Press, Cambridge.

Meuret, J-L. (1992) *The FISA Centenary Book*. Fédération Internationale des Sociétés d'Aviron, Oberhofen am Thunersee.

Chapter 2
Biomechanics

V. Kleshnev

Gearing

In sports such as rowing and cycling the term "gearing" is used for the ratio of the velocity of locomotion to that of the athlete's movement. According to the lever law, the ratio of forces is inversely proportional to the ratio of velocities. Athletes therefore have to apply proportionally more force as the gearing decreases the velocity of their action at constant speed of locomotion. In rowing, gearing is defined by two main variables: the length of the oar versus its inboard length (Fig. 2.1).

The oar length is measured from the handle top to the outer edge of the blade in the line of the shaft. The inboard length is measured from the handle top to the face of the button. However, the resultant forces are applied at different points of the blade:

• The point of the handle force application is difficult to locate and it may vary among rowers. We assume that the handle force is applied at the center of the handle, which is located 6 cm from the handle top in sculling and 15 cm from the top in sweep rowing.

• The gate force is applied on the center of the pin, which offsets from the button on the half width of the gate and it is usually 2 cm.

• The blade force is applied at the center of water pressure on the blade. This force is even more difficult to define than the force on the handle and it may vary depending on the angle of the oar relative to the boat. We assume that it is applied at the geo- metric center of the blade, which is usually located 20 cm from the blade's outer edge in sculling and 25 cm from the edge in sweep rowing.

Gearing is heavier in sculling than in sweep boats. The variation between small and large boats is small and does not correspond to the difference in the speed of the boat (Table 2.1). The difference in the handle speeds between 1×/2- and 4×/8+ is quite significant (12–14%). This leads to the variation of the racing rate, which varies from 34–36 strokes·min^{-1} in 1×/2- to 39–40 strokes·min^{-1} in 4×/8+.

Actual gearing is heavier at the catch and finish of the drive than at the perpendicular position of the oar. At the catch, and at the finish, the blade moves in an angle relative to the boat movement and its longitudinal component is equal to cosine of the angle (e.g., at a catch angle of 60°, the gearing is two times heavier and at 45° it is 30% heavier than at the perpendicular oar position).

The workplace

It is important to set up the rower's workplace properly, because its geometry affects vectors of forces and velocities and hence efficiency and effectiveness of the rowing technique (Fig. 2.2).

• Gate height is measured from seat to the bottom of the oarlock and it varies from 14 to 19 cm depending on the rower's height. In sculling, the left gate is usually 0.5–2 cm higher than the right in order to allow the hands to pass above each other when the oars are perpendicular to the boat.

Table 2.1 Oar gearing (Nolte, 2005) and corresponding speed characteristics (World best times for 2006) in different boat types.

Boat type	Oar length (m)	Inboard (m)	Actual inboard (m)	Actual outboard (m)	Actual gearing	Boat speed Men (m·s⁻¹)	Boat speed Women (m·s⁻¹)	Handle speed Men (m·s⁻¹)	Handle speed Women (m·s⁻¹)
1×	2.88	0.88	0.84	1.78	2.119	5.05	4.68	2.38	2.21
2×	2.88	0.88	0.84	1.78	2.119	5.49	5.02	2.59	2.37
4×	2.89	0.875	0.835	1.795	2.150	5.92	5.39	2.76	2.51
2−	3.72	1.16	1.03	2.29	2.223	5.34	4.83	2.40	2.17
4−	3.73	1.15	1.02	2.31	2.265	5.86		2.59	
8+	3.73	1.14	1.01	2.32	2.297	6.25	5.61	2.72	2.44

1×, single sculls; 2×, double sculls; 4×, quadruple sculls; 2−, coxless pair; 4−, coxless four; 8+, coxed eight.

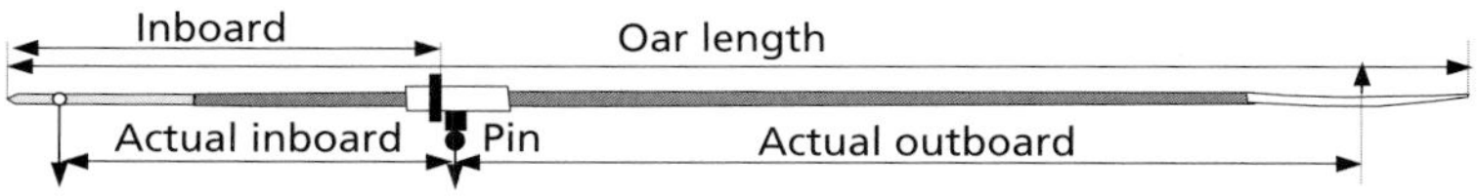

Fig. 2.1 Oar gearing variables.

Fig. 2.2 Variables of the rower's workplace geometry.

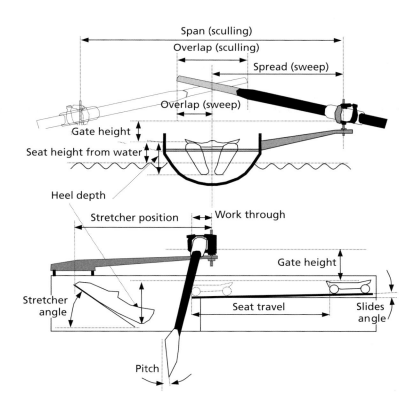

• The heel depth is measured from seat to the bottom of the shoes and varies from 15 to 22 cm depending on the rower's body proportions.

• The seat height from water varies depending on boat type and weight of the rowers.

• The span in sculling is measured from pin to pin. In sweep rowing, the spread is measured from pin to the boat centerline. Usually, the inboard length is longer than the spread in sweep boats or half of the span in sculling boats. This makes overlap measured between tops of the handles in sculling, which is usually 15–20 cm, and between the boat centerline and top of the handle in sweep rowing of 25–30 cm.

• The stretcher position is measured from the pin to the toes of the shoes and is 50–65 cm.

• The "work through" is the distance from the pin to the end of the slides and is 5–12 cm.

• The distance that the seat travels is usually 60–65 cm.

• The stretcher angle varies from 36° to 45°.

• The slide angle is usually set between 0.5° and 1.5°.

• The oar pitch is the angle between the vertical line and the blade. The angle depends on two settings: the pitch of the blade relative to the sleeve and the gate pitch. The pitch of the blade is usually set to zero and the gate pitch varies between 2° and 6°. If the pin is leaning inwards, then the pitch at the catch will be less and at the finish more than the pitch at the perpendicular position of the oar. Conversely, an outward leaning of the pin produces the opposite changes. Usually, the pin is set vertically, but some coaches use 1–2° outward leaning of the pin, which prevents the blade from going too deep at the catch and too shallow at the finish of the drive.

Mechanics

Propulsion and blade efficiency

When the rower applies force to the oar handle (F_h), it is transferred to the blade and produces pressure on the water. According to Newton's third law this force creates a reaction force on the blade (F_b), which is the force that accelerates the rower–boat–oars system (RBOS) forward (Fig. 2.3). During the drive phase, the center of mass (CM) of the whole system moves forward and the center of pressure (CP) of the oar slips through the water. Some point on the oar shaft remains stationary and can be considered as an imaginary fulcrum. This fulcrum is not a real fulcrum because there is no support at this point (Fig. 2.4). The position of the fulcrum changes during the drive phase and depends on the blade

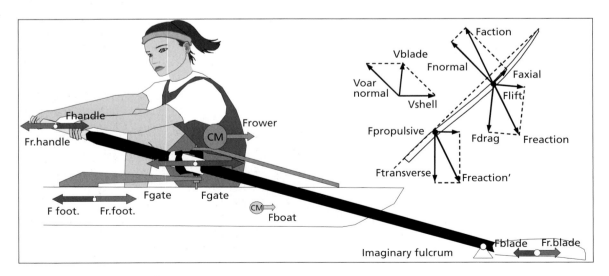

Fig. 2.3 Forces in the rower–boat–oar system.

propulsive efficiency: the higher the efficiency, the closer the fulcrum to the CP of the blade. The fulcrum coincides with CP at 100% efficiency.

The reaction force on the blade is the sum of the drag and the lift forces. As the angle of the oar relative to the boat changes through the drive, the ratio of the drag and lift forces changes from 1:2 at the catch (60°) to 1:0 at the perpendicular position (Caplan and Gardner, 2005). The lift force does not result in any loss of energy (i.e., it is 100% efficient) because the vectors of force and velocity are perpendicular to each other. The vector of the drag force is parallel to the velocity vector and has an opposite direction.

Waste of energy is calculated as a scalar (dot) product of blade force and velocity vectors. Propulsive power is the product of the force and velocity vectors applied to the CM of RBOS. The sum of the propulsive and the waste posers equals the total power applied to the oar handle. Propulsive efficiency of the blade is a ratio of the propulsive power to the total power.

Propulsive efficiency of the blade can be derived by means of measuring the instantaneous boat velocity, oar angle and a force at the oar handle or gate. F_b is calculated using handle force and oar gearing. The blade velocity (vb) is derived using oar angle and boat velocity data.

Propulsive efficiency of the blade depends on the relative pressure on the blade (i.e., the ratio of the blade force to its area). Lower pressure relates to less slippage of the blade through the water and higher blade propulsive efficiency. Thus, efficiency can be increased by reducing blade force or increasing blade area. The blade force is reduced at the same handle force by increasing the oar gearing ratio (shorter inboard and longer outboard distance). However, very heavy gearing will decrease muscular efficiency, because the handle speed will decrease and that makes the muscles work in a slow static-like fashion.

An increase of the blade area is also limited because a wider blade takes more time and requires more effort for entry and extraction from the water. A very long blade is also inefficient, because it can create counter-movement effect on the backside of the blade. Also, the blade efficiency is affected by the velocity of the boat and it is higher in faster (bigger) boat types. Sculling has higher blade efficiency than sweep rowing, which can be explained by the higher sum of the blade area. This could be one of the reasons why sculling boats are faster than sweep boats of the same size.

Characteristics of the force application affect blade efficiency and may be controlled by the rower. A force curve with a peak increases blade slippage and decreases efficiency. Conversely, a rectangular shape of the force curve affects efficiency positively. There is a moderate correlation between the ratio of average to maximal force, taken as a measure of the shape of the force curve (100% for rectangle, 50% for triangle), and blade efficiency ($r = 0.48$; $P < 0.01$).

Bigger boats have higher blade efficiency because of higher average speed, which makes the lift force more significant (Table 2.2). Scullers are efficient

Table 2.2 Blade propulsive efficiency in Olympic rowing events.

Boat type	Men Heavy (%)	Light (%)	Woman Heavy (%)	Light (%)	Average (%)
1×	79.6		78.5		79.0
2−	78.5		80.6		79.4
2×	82.3	81.9	83.6	84.1	83.0
4−	80.2	82.1	80.5		81.0
4×	83.7		87.3		85.5
8−	81.4		81.5		81.4

1×, single sculls; 2×, double sculls; 4×, quadruple sculls; 2−, coxless pair; 4−, coxless four; 8−, coxless eight.

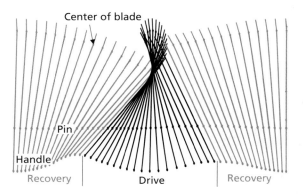

Fig. 2.4 Path of the oar during the stroke cycle.

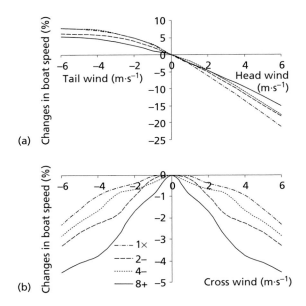

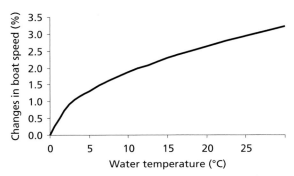

Fig. 2.6 Boat speed at different water temperature (Filter, 2000).

Fig. 2.5 Boat speed at (a) straight and (b) cross winds (Filter, 2000).

because of the larger total area of the blade. Higher blade efficiency in lightweight women's crews can be explained by lower force application, which relates to lower relative pressure on the blade and less slippage through the water.

The Vortex Edge "big blade" was introduced in an attempt to increase efficiency (Concept 2 website). The overall improvement of the blade efficiency with Vortex is about 2%. Application of the Vortex shifts the center of pressure towards the outer edge of the blade, which is equivalent to increasing the outboard lever of the oar.

Boat speed

According to fluid dynamics the drag resistance force is proportional to the square of boat speed and the drag power is proportional to the cube of the velocity. Therefore, in order to increase the speed of the boat twofold, a fourfold higher drag force has to be overcome and an eightfold higher power needs to be applied.

Normally, the hydrodynamic resistance of the water represents 85% of the total drag force, which includes 70% water friction, 10% wave resistance and 5% pressure resistance. Aerodynamic resistance represents ~15%, but in head wind of $5\,m\cdot s^{-1}$ it increases to 30% and at wind speed of $10\,m\cdot s^{-1}$ represents 50% of the total drag. Correspondingly, in tail wind equal to the boat speed air resistance is eliminated (Fig. 2.5). The body of the rower creates approximately 75% of air resistance, the oars represent nearly 20% and the remaining 5% depends on the boat hull and the riggers. Straight head wind is beneficial for big boats, because the bow rower shields the rest of the crew, which decreases the drag. Cross-head wind has less influence on small boats (Fig. 2.5b).

Water viscosity decreases at higher water temperature, which decreases hydrodynamic resistance and allows higher boat speeds (Fig. 2.6).

Because of the periodic nature of the drive phase in rowing, the boat speed varies during the stroke cycle (Fig. 2.7a). The drag power increases more at a higher than average boat velocity (dash shaded area) than it is reduced at a lower than average velocity (cross shaded area). The total energy expenditure at variable boat velocity is therefore higher compared with constant velocity.

The ratio of the minimal power required to propel the boat at a given speed to the actual propulsive power at variable boat velocity is called "boat efficiency."

For improvement of the boat's efficiency, Sanderson and Martindale (1986) suggested optimization of the rowers' movement on recovery to maintain

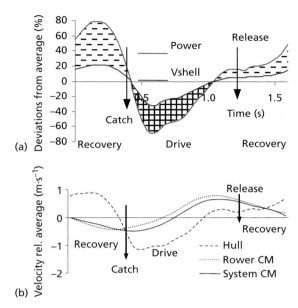

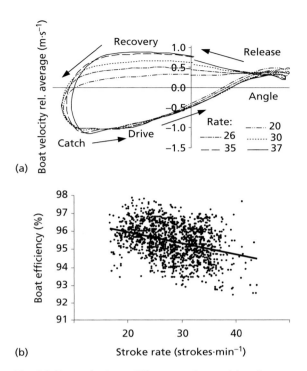

Fig. 2.7 Deviations of the shell velocity and drag power from average (a); relative velocities of the hull, rowers and RBOS centers of mass (b).

Fig. 2.8 Boat velocity at different stroke rate (a) and dependence boat efficiency on the stroke rate (b).

Table 2.3 Boat efficiency of rowing in Olympic boat types.

| Boat type | Men | | Woman | | |
	Heavy (%)	Light (%)	Heavy (%)	Light (%)	Average (%)
1×	95.1		94.5		94.8
2–	94.9		95.1		95.0
2×	94.9	95.5	95.4	96.3	95.5
4×	96.2		95.6		95.9
4–	95.4	95.3	91.9		94.2
8+	96.4		96.5		96.4

1×, single sculls; 2×, double sculls; 4×, quadruple sculls; 2–, coxless pair; 4–, coxless four; 8+, coxed eight.

the shell speed as constant as possible (Table 2.3). At high stroke rates, the recovery time is shorter and that dictates faster movement of the rowers' mass and higher acceleration of the shell. Therefore, the boat velocity fluctuations increase with stroke rate (Fig. 2.8a), which leads to a decrease of the boat

velocity efficiency (Fig. 2.8b) and stroke rate has a negative correlation with the boat efficiency ($r = -0.34$; $P < 0.05$). On average, the boat's efficiency drops 1.4% from a stroke rate of 20 (96.0%) to 40 (94.6%).

Newton's laws of motion

The implication of Newton's first law is that rowers have to apply force to overcome drag and maintain linear movement of the boat. When force is applied to the blade during the drive phase, an equal and opposite directed reaction force is created, according to Newton's third law. The forward component of this reaction force is the reason for acceleration of the boat–oar–rower center of mass. According to Newton's second law, the magnitude of this acceleration is proportional to the mass of the system and the magnitude of the propulsive force. When the center of mass of the boat accelerates, it accumulates kinetic energy, which is spent on overcoming drag resistance and lost as heat to the surroundings of the boat.

However, rowing mechanics is not simple. It may appear that the main goal of the crew is acceleration of the boat and because the rowers sit in the boat that system moves as fast as the boat does. This simplistic observation leads to erroneous coaching theories, which can harm performance in rowing when it is advised to maximize handle gate force in order to accelerate the boat and, at the same time, minimize the force on the foot-stretcher, because it pushes the boat backwards.

The following steps help to understand the principles of effective rowing technique:

1 To increase the boat speed, rowers have to expend more power to overcome higher drag resistance ($P = kv^3$).

2 The kinetic energy of the whole boat–rower system can be increased (accumulated) only during the drive phase. The increase of the shell's velocity during the recovery is explained by the transfer of the crew's kinetic energy.

3 Because the crew's mass is larger than that of the boat, the crew accumulates 5–6 times more kinetic energy than the boat ($Ek = mv^2/2$). Therefore, the main target for an effective drive phase is to increase the velocity of the crew's center of mass.

4 The only force that accelerates the rower's center of mass forward is the reaction force on the stretcher. Therefore, maximizing of the stretcher force is the main target of the drive. Conversely, the handle force pulls the rower backwards.

5 To apply a high stretcher force is not enough for a rower's acceleration. The stretcher must have a supporting connection to the water through the rigger and oar.

6 The stretcher (and the whole shell) has to move fast forwards at the moment of the leg drive.

Rowing can, accordingly, be considered as a series of jumps, where each drive phase is a jump and recovery represents the flight phase. With this consideration, longer jumps or a higher jump frequency result in higher rowing speed. The major difference between rowing and jumping is that rowers have to create support on the stretcher by placing the blade in the water and applying handle force.

Timing of the stroke cycle

Temporal or phase analysis has an important role in sport biomechanics and is the most versatile biomechanical method of analysis across different sports. Methods based on mechanical parameters (position, velocity, force, etc.) are very different in various sport motions. The phase analysis is based on time only and can represent different motions as a sequence of phases and subphases.

Accelerations of the boat–rower system center of mass as well as the oar and seat velocity are used for definition of the microphases of the stroke cycle (Fig. 2.9). Figure 2.10 shows biomechanical parameters of a single sculler. Six microphases of the drive phase (D1–D6) and three microphases of the recovery (R1, R2, R3) are defined in Table 2.4.

Between D1 and D2 the rower pushes to accelerate their body mass and decelerate the boat because he or she has to change direction of movement from the stern to bow at the catch. The quicker the D1–D2 are, the better. During D3 the rower accelerates the boat to create faster moving support on the foot-stretcher to further accelerate his or her body. D3 is important for an effective drive phase but in some crews this phase is absent. Fast increasing of the handle force is the main condition of its presence.

During D4 the rower pushes the stretcher again to accelerate and accumulates the main part of kinetic energy. Effectiveness of this phase depends on the amount of gained boat speed during D3 and fast powerful leg drive. The final boat acceleration microphases D5 and D6 utilize more pull by means of the trunk and the work of the arms. Forces and total system acceleration decrease during this phase and acceleration of the rower becomes negative transferring kinetic energy to the boat. This push–pull–push–pull coordination during the drive requires coordination and "boat feel" from the rowers.

Biomechanical variables

Rowing provides an excellent model for biomechanical measurements. The first of such measurements were carried out by Atkinson in 1896. Since then, biomechanical measurements have become common practice both for research and athlete

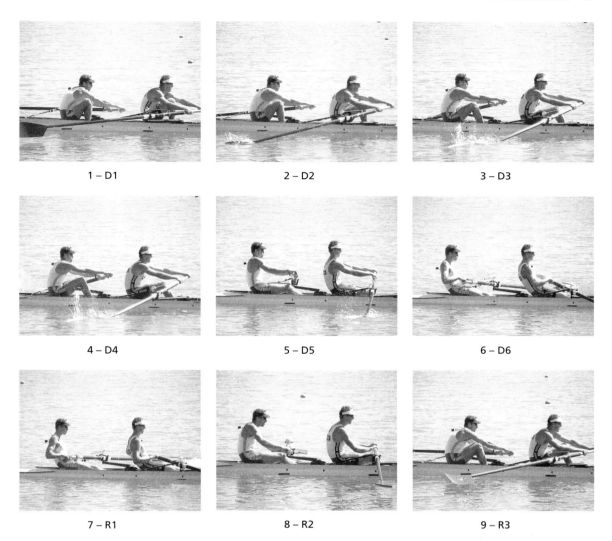

Fig. 2.9 Microphases of the stroke cycle (key event and the following phase). Men's pair James Tomkins and Drew Ginn, Olympic Champions of Athens Games 2004. Stroke rate 36.5 strokes·min⁻¹, video 25 frames·s⁻¹, frame number, microphase.

training purposes. The main variables for rowing biomechanics are the oar angle, force application, boat velocity and acceleration, and body segments' movement.

Oar angle

The horizontal oar angle defines the amplitude of the rower's movement. The angle is measured from the perpendicular position of the oar relative to the boat axis, which defines zero degree. The catch angle is defined as the minimal negative angle and the release angle is the maximal positive angle. The horizontal oar angle is used for definition of the start of the stroke cycle, which occurs at zero oar angle during recovery (Table 2.5) (Kleshnev, 2005). The total rowing angle can be 4% longer at a low stroke rate of 20–24 strokes·min⁻¹.

A vertical oar angle is useful for defining of the rower's oar handling skills. It reads zero degree when

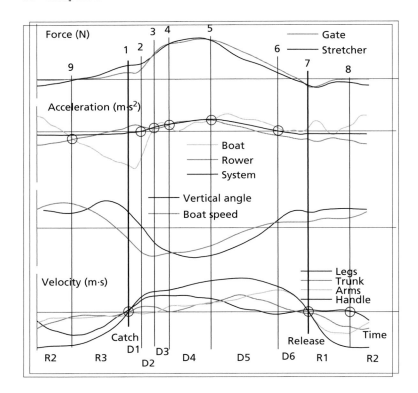

Fig. 2.10 Biomechanical parameters and microphases of the stroke cycle (M1×, rate 32 strokes·min⁻¹). Key events are marked with circles.

the center of the blade is at the water level and negative downwards.

Forces

The forces in rowing are usually measured at the handle and at the gate (pin).

The handle force can be determined by means of measuring the bend of oar shaft. The point of the handle force application is not certain, especially in sweep rowing, where the rower can pull more with the inside or the outside arm. This can create a problem if the ambition is to know the handle force itself, but it produces more reliable values of rowing power applied to the handle, because it is calculated using the moment of force.

The gate force is measured using instrumented gates. This method produces more accurate and informative data on the force applied to the boat, but calculation of the power from the gate force is not accurate (Table 2.6).

The graph of the force relative to time or horizontal oar angle is called the "force curve," which is an indicator of rowing technique. Peak force develops earlier in big fast boats and at a higher stroke rate.

Body segments input

On average, each of three body segments contributes approximately one-third to the total length of the stroke arc (legs a bit more, trunk a bit less). The legs execute their work during the first half of the drive, when the force exertion is maximal. Therefore, the legs produce nearly half of the rowing power (46%); the trunk produces nearly one-third (32%) and arms a little more than one-fifth (22%) (Kleshnev, 2000). At higher stroke rates the legs increase their percentage contribution to power. Thus, trunk muscles utilize only about 55% of their work capacity during rowing. At the same time, the arms use about 75% and the legs up to 95% of their respective work capacity.

Rowing technique

Rowing styles and efficiency

Rowing styles are defined by movement of the two biggest body segments: the legs and the trunk. The most popular attempt to classify rowing styles was

Table 2.4 Microphases and key events of the stroke cycle.

No.	Key event	Microphase ID	Microphase
1	Catch, beginning of the drive. Oar changes direction of movement	D1. Blade immersion	Acceleration is negative. Small inertial forces are applied to the handle and the gate, but the foot-stretcher force is significant. This produces a negative peak of the boat's acceleration and a positive peak acceleration of the rower's center of mass. There is a fast increase of the handle and leg speed
2	Acceleration becomes positive. The center of the blade crosses the water level	D2. Initial acceleration of the rower	Handle force increases, which leads to the gain of the boat's acceleration, but it is still negative and lower than the rowers' center of mass acceleration
3	Acceleration of the boat becomes higher than the rowers' center of mass acceleration. This is caused by the increase of the gate force, which becomes higher than the stretcher force	D3. Initial boat acceleration	First positive peak of the boat's acceleration and cavity of the rower's acceleration. The blade is fully immersed. Maximal speed of the legs
4	Acceleration of the boat decreases and becomes lower than the rower's acceleration. This is caused by the increase of the stretcher force, which again becomes higher than the gate force	D4. Acceleration of the rower	The rower–system accelerations increase slowly. Handle speed continues to grow. Legs speed decreases and trunk speed increases
5	Boat acceleration again becomes higher than the rowers' center of mass acceleration. This is caused by a decrease in the foot-stretcher force, which becomes lower than the gate force	D5. Boat acceleration	All forces are decreasing, but the foot-stretcher force is decreasing faster than the gate force, which produces the highest boat acceleration. The rower's and system's acceleration decrease. The oar crosses perpendicular to the boat. The handle and trunk achieve their maximal speed.
6	The system's acceleration becomes negative. The center of the blade crosses the water level	D6. Blade removal	The handle continues to move towards the bow. The arms achieve the maximal speed. The rower's mass begins the recovery phase (negative acceleration). Nearly zero boat acceleration
7	Release, end of the drive. The oar handle movement changes direction toward the stern	R1. Arms and trunk return	The moment of inertia transfers from the rower's upper body to the boat mass. This causes a quick positive peak of boat acceleration and negative rower's acceleration
8	The seat starts moving toward the stern. Rowers cause an increase of the boat's acceleration and a quicker decrease of the rowers' center of mass acceleration	R2. Legs return	The boat acceleration is positive (depending on the stroke rate), but rower's and system accelerations are negative. The leg speed towards the stern is increasing. Arms are nearly straight, trunk crosses the vertical position
9	Rower starts pushing foot-stretcher. The speed of the seat decreases and boat acceleration becomes negative	R3. Catch preparation	Rowers push the stretcher stronger. This causes boat deceleration, but center of mass of the rowers starts acceleration. Arms and oars prepare for the blade entry to the water

by Klavora (1977), which defines the following three main styles.

1 The **Rosenberg** style is named after Allen Rosenberg, who was the head coach of many USA national rowing teams 1961–76. This is the most traditional style and inherits development in technique introduced by the great English–Australian coach Steve Fairbairn at the end of 19th and early decades of the 20th century. This style is characterized by large forward declination of the trunk at the beginning of the stroke followed by strong leg extension without significant trunk activation. At the end of the cycle the trunk stops in the deep backward position.

2 The **Adam** style was developed in the 1960s by the innovative coach Carl Adam from West Germany. This style has a comparatively long leg drive, limited amplitude of the trunk and simultaneous activity of legs and trunk during the stroke.

3 The **DDR** style was developed by coaches and scientists of East Germany—the most successful rowing nation in the 1970s. The style is characterized by large forward declination of the trunk, which begins the drive, followed by simultaneous activity of the legs.

Two main factors that distinguish these styles are timing (simultaneous or consequent activity of two biggest body segments) and emphasis during the drive (on legs or trunk). These factors can be illustrated as x and y axes of a quadrant (Fig. 2.11).

These three styles perfectly fit three-quarters of the quadrant. However, a fourth rowing style exists. This style has consequent timing and emphasis on the legs drive. This style is called the "**Grinko** style"

after the Russian coach Igor Grinko who coached World Champions M4× of USSR and then 1990 World Champion and 2004 Silver Olympic medalist in M1× Jueri Jaanson. This style inherits the traditions of the USSR school of rowing technique, which produced great rowers from 1950–60 including three times Olympic champion Viacheslav Ivanov (see Fig. 1.25).

The rowing style correlates with the shape of force curve, which affects the amount of power generated and blade propulsive efficiency. A sequenced work of the legs and trunk (Rosenberg and Grinko rowing styles) usually produces a triangular shape of the force curve and higher peak force and power values (Fig. 2.12). This leads to higher slippage of the blade through the water which causes energy losses. Lower blade propulsive efficiency, however, can be more than compensated for by higher values of force and power produced per kilogram of body weight. Active use of the trunk produces even more

Table 2.5 Average oar angles in different categories of rowers at racing stroke rate.

Categories	Catch angle	Release angle (°)	Total angle (°)
Men scull	−66.5	43.8	110.4
Men light scull	−64.5	42.6	107.1
Men sweep	−56.8	34.3	91.2
Men light sweep	−54.3	33.6	87.9
Women scull	−62.2	43.0	105.2
Women light scull	−61.3	42.8	104.2
Women sweep	−53.5	33.4	86.9

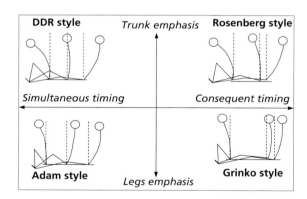

Fig. 2.11 Quadrant of rowing styles.

Table 2.6 The handle forces and rowing power at racing rate in different categories of rowers.

Rower's categories	Maximal handle force (N)	Average force during the drive (N)	Rowing power (W)
Men scull	766	405	528
Men light scull	692	360	464
Men sweep	671	331	520
Men light sweep	590	294	425
Women scull	547	286	329
Women light scull	477	253	285
Women sweep	479	238	308

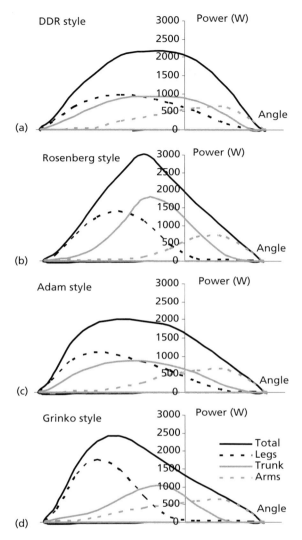

Fig. 2.12 Effect of the segments sequence and emphasis on the shape of power curve.

power and the Rosenberg style can be considered as the most powerful rowing style.

Simultaneous work of the legs and trunk (the two German rowing styles) produces a more rectangular shape of the force curve, but the peak force and power are lower (Fig. 2.12b). More even pressure on the blade improves its propulsive efficiency. However, the slower and more static character of the legs and trunk work does not allow delivery of its optimal power.

Emphasis of legs or trunk work affects the position of the peak force and power. Styles with legs emphasis (Adam and Grinko styles) allow quicker increase of the force and earlier peak of the force curve. This increases the initial boat acceleration (D3), improves the temporal structure of the drive and makes it more effective.

Styles with trunk emphasis (Rosenberg and DDR styles) produce more power because of better use of big muscle groups such as the gluteus and longissimus muscles. However, these muscles are congenitally slow because they are intended to maintain body posture. This fact, together with the significant mass of the torso, does not allow for a quick increase of the force and shift the peak of the force curve closer to the middle of the drive, making the temporal structure of the drive less effective.

However, it is uncommon that these rowing styles are found in their pure form. Most rowers adopt a hybrid style between these four extremes. The choice of style depends on many factors such as the body structure of the rower. For example, it is unlikely that rowers with short legs will adopt a style that emphasizes the importance of a long slide.

Coordination, coaching and feedback

Rowing looks quite simple but in fact it requires a very high level of coordination and sophisticated motor control. The rower has to coordinate his or her body movement along with the oar's three-dimensional movement and to maintain the balance of the boat. The task becomes even more complicated in crews, where each rower has to synchronize his or her movement with that of other members of the crew.

Because of the short time of the drive phase (<1 s) and the fast movement of big muscle groups, rowers cannot change movement pattern during the drive. They can only evaluate their sensations after completion of each stroke and make corrections for the next one.

The coach watches the crew and compares his or her impression with an ideal model of rowing technique. The coach then provides verbal feedback to the rowers more or less immediately: after each stroke, after completion of a bout of training, after a session, a day or a week. A good coach also asks for feedback from the athletes which helps him or her to evaluate the effectiveness of the actions and to find better methods for correcting technique.

Several technical tools have become popular for providing feedback to rowers and coaches:

- StrokeCoach and SpeedCoach™ provide immediate feedback on stroke rate and boat speed.
- Visual feedback can include videotape and replay after the session or in immediate mode using a personal head-mounted display.
- Biomechanical data acquisition systems can measure the force applied by the rower, oar angles and other mechanical parameters (seat and trunk position, etc.).

Such equipment looks attractive and it is powerful for correction of rowing technique. It is, however, necessary to understand what needs to be corrected and in what direction. Proper theory of rowing biomechanics is crucial when using technical methods of rowing technique correction.

References

Atkinson, E. (1896) A rowing indicator. *Natural Science* **8**, 178.

Caplan, N. & Gardner, T.N. (2005) A new measurement system for the determination of oar blade forces in rowing. In: M.H. Hamza, ed. *Proceedings of the 3rd IASTed International Conference on Biomechanics*. Acta Press, Calgary, Canada.

Concept 2 website. http://www.concept2.com/05/oars/vortex1.asp

Filter, K. (2000) Effect of wind on boat speed. Materials of FISA coaches conference in Seville.

Klavora, P. (1977) Three predominant styles: the Adam style; the DDR style; the Rosenberg style. *Catch (Ottawa)* **9**, 13.

Kleshnev, V. (2000) Power in rowing. *Proceedings of XVIII Congress of ISBS, Hong Kong*, Vol. II, pp. 662–666.

Kleshnev, V. (2005) Technology for technique improvement. In: V. Nolte, ed. *Rowing Faster*. Human Kinetics, Champaign, IL. pp. 209–228.

Nolte, V. (2005) Rigging. In: V. Nolte, ed. *Rowing Faster*. Human Kinetics, Champaign, IL. pp. 125–140.

Sanderson, B. & Martindale, W. (1986) Towards optimizing rowing technique. *Medicine and Science in Sports and Exercise* **18**, 454–468.

Chapter 3
The oarsman

J. Jürimäe, T. Jürimäe and J. Maestu

Introduction

Among sport disciplines the differences in physical and physiologic characteristics of elite athletes represent heredity while physical training, nutrition and sociocultural factors are also important. Elite athletes are selected and train for the physical and physiologic requirements of the sport. Rowing is characterized as a strength and endurance sport and performance depends on specific kinanthropometric, physiologic, psychologic, technical and tactical capacities. Cooperation with other team members also has an important role. In addition to the 2000 m competition, competitions are held for distances from 200 and 500 m to 4 and 10 km. However, this chapter focuses on the physical profile that characterizes rowing over the classic 2000 m distance.

Physical requirements

The rowing stroke is supported by the sliding seat so that the drive phase is sequentially performed by extension of the legs and extension of the trunk with simultaneous flexion of the arms. The contributing role of the arms is minor in absolute force production but critical for efficiency. Successful elite rowers produce about 75–80% of their power with their legs and 20–25% with their arms. The trunk muscles form a tight link between the feet on the stretcher and the oar — to ensure that the force generated by the legs is most efficiently carried to the oar handle. To produce an effective stroke, the rower has to achieve a combination of high stroke force and optimal stroke length. These requirements tend to select rowers of a specific body size, shape and morphology.

Body build

Rowing is a weight-supported sport and anthropometric data of elite adult rowers emphasize the importance of the body mass and size. Successful open class rowers are as lean, but much heavier and taller, with long arms and a tall sitting height compared with athletes in other endurance sport disciplines. Long arms are helpful in obtaining an adequate stroke length. Because rowing is a strength endurance sport, in which body mass and body size are performance-related factors, lightweight rowing has been introduced. The physical characteristics of lightweight rowers differ from open class rowers, with the lightweight rower being more similar to untrained controls.

The successful elite male open class rower is approximately 195 cm tall and weighs about 95 kg, while the desired height and weight of the elite open class female rower is 182 cm and 80 kg, respectively. Over the last 30 years, the height and weight of elite rowers has not changed much, indicating that the rigorous process of selection of the team has had little influence on the progressive improvement in rowing performance. Yet the winners of international regattas are usually about 10% taller and 25% heavier than a normative reference sample. Furthermore, the gold medal winners are consistently taller and heavier than national champions. Because the mentioned heights and weights required for competitive success are less likely to be found among African, Asian and Latin American nations, the lightweight rowing classification is justified. Successful lightweight males average about 184 cm, while lightweight females have a height of about 170 cm. The physical trait in lightweight rowers has remained stable for the past two decades and continues to be a determinant of competitive success. Lightweight rowers are at a mechanical advantage if they are tall and have long legs. There is a trend for successful lightweight rowers to become taller and even more slender as, in order to meet the weight limitation, height comes at the expense of fat and other soft tissue mass. World Championship lightweight medalists occasionally weigh less than non-medalists, with higher values for different length, breadth and girth dimensions. Sweep rowers in open class are consistently taller and heavier than scullers, amounting to 2 cm and 4 kg for men, and 3 cm and 3 kg for women. The reason why sweep rowers are heavier, taller and more muscular than scullers may be a result of the dynamics of boat movement. Boats with sweep oars on average involve more athletes and a coxswain in the coxed pair, four and eight. The weight of the coxswain imposes a greater deceleration of the boat at the catch of the stroke, where the blade enters the water and force is applied to the oar, because of the change of the direction of the bodies in the boat and a high force is required to accelerate the boat. Thus, tall, muscular and heavy rowers are favored.

Growth and development of successful rowers

The height of male rowers at age 16 is about 187 cm and the average body mass is about 80 kg. Until the end of growth, around age 19, height increases about 10 cm and weight increases about 15 kg. Both male and female rowers are already tall in early childhood, and they maintain their relative characteristics throughout adolescence. These trends suggest no effect of regular training on growth in body size. Because physique is an important element of performance in rowing and determines the adaptability to prolonged training, quantification of physique in junior rowers may be used in evaluating models for talent identification. The 383 male and 245 female junior participants of the 1997 World Junior Rowing Championships were studied by Bourgois *et al.* (1998) to establish a rowing specific anthropometric profile. Male junior rowers are 7% taller and 27% heavier than a normative reference group. The mean height of elite junior male rowers varies between 187 and 192 cm, which is quite similar to the adult open class rowers (185–195 cm). However, adult open class rowers are heavier (85–95 kg) than the elite junior rowers (81–84 kg). When compared with lightweight rowers, elite male junior rowers are on average 7 cm taller and 12 kg heavier than male lightweight rowers. Female elite junior rowers are also 7% taller and 25% heavier when compared with a normative reference group. The mean height (175–177 cm) and weight (70–72 kg) are within the range of values obtained for adult open class female rowers (173–18 cm and 67–76 kg). The elite junior female rowers are on average 6.7 cm taller and 11.9 kg heavier than the female lightweight rowers. Junior male and female rowers seem to have a lower sitting height relative to stature when compared with a normative reference group and adult open class rowers, while there are no differences between junior and lightweight rowers.

Elite junior male rowers have greater length, breadth and girth dimensions than the general population and lightweight rowers, but these values are lower than open class rowers. Similarly, the elite junior female rowers have greater length dimensions, and greater breadths and girths than a reference group and lightweight rowers but similar values to senior open class rowers (Table 3.1). The most able young rowers can be distinguished by their height, skeletal robustness and muscular development. This is evident when anthropometric characteristics of finalists in junior male and female rowers are compared with the rowers who do not make the finals (Table 3.2). The finalists are heavier and taller, with higher values for most length,

Table 3.1 Comparison of mean body dimensions of international male and female rowers (Bourgois *et al.* 1998).

Body dimensions	Open class males (*n* = 65)	Lightweight males (*n* = 144)	Junior males (*n* = 383)	Open class females (*n* = 51)	Lightweight females (*n* = 50)	Junior females (*n* = 220)
Age (years)	24.2	24.3	17.8	23.8	24.1	17.5
Stature (cm)	191.3	180.7	187.4	174.3	167.1	174.5
Body mass (kg)	90	70.3	82.2	67.4	57.1	69.5
Sitting height (cm)	99.7	93.8	96.8	92.1	87.6	90.8
Leg length (cm)	91.7	87.6	90.7	82.3	81.2	83.9
SHSR (%)	52.1	51.5	51.6	52.8	52.4	52.0
LLSR (%)	47.9	48.5	48.4	47.2	48.6	48.1
Biceps girth (cm)	–	30.7	32.9	29.3	26.2	29.0
Thigh girth (cm)	60.3	51.0	57.9	57.5	49.2	58.5
Triceps skinfold (mm)	8.4	5.5	7.9	14.6	10.0	14.0
Subscapular skinfold (mm)	8.7	8.0	8.9	9.1	8.5	10.2
Thigh skinfold (mm)	10.8	8.0	11.5	21.5	17.6	22.3
Calf skinfold (mm)	6.3	5.4	8.4	12.8	11.3	16.0
Sum of skinfolds (mm)	34.2	26.9	36.7	58.0	47.4	62.5

LLSR, leg length to stature ratio; SHSR, sitting height to stature ratio.

Table 3.2 Comparison of mean body dimensions among male and female junior rowers by performance: finalists and non-finalists (Bourgois *et al.* 1998).

Body dimensions	Male finalists (*n* = 144)	Male non-finalists (*n* = 222)	Female finalists (*n* = 112)	Female non-finalists (*n* = 94)
Stature (cm)	189.3	186.3	176.6	172.7
Body mass (kg)	84.8	80.6	71.3	67.7
Sitting height (cm)	97.6	96.2	91.6	90.1
Leg length (cm)	91.6	90.1	85.1	82.6
SHSR (%)	51.6	51.6	51.9	52.2
LLSR (%)	48.4	48.4	48.2	47.8
Biceps girth (cm)	33.5	32.6	29.3	28.7
Thigh girth (cm)	58.7	57.5	59.2	57.8

LLSR, leg length to stature ratio; SHSR, sitting height to stature ratio.

breadth and girth dimensions. It is therefore advantageous for the rower to be tall and heavy, while long arms and legs are particularly helpful in giving extra leverage. In addition, large rowers have a greater cross-sectional area of muscle and a greater absolute metabolic capacity.

Regular training is of importance for a late mean age at menarche. Results from the participants of the 1997 World Junior Rowing Championships reveal that the mean age at menarche of rowers is 12.8 years and that is not different from a non-athletic reference population. However, delayed mean age at menarche is seen in female junior rowers who started their rowing training before compared with those who started their rowing training after menarche, with mean ages of 13.4 and 12.4 years, respectively. This observation suggests that the later age at menarche observed in elite junior rowers who began their rowing training before menarche is a consequence of the intense routine prepubertal physical exercise. However, such conclusions should be taken cautiously as no differences can be demonstrated for chronologic age or any body compositional variables. No longitudinal data on rowing athletes are available. It can be suggested that girls active in rowing present a pattern of growth and maturation characteristics similar to average maturing individuals, but they are taller and heavier than the reference population and therefore there is no evidence to indicate that intense rowing training has a negative influence on the maturation of female rowers.

Body composition

Resistance to the forward movement of the boat is approximately proportional to two-thirds of the power of the weight of the vessel and its crew members. With the exception of lightweight competitions, it is advantageous to recruit rowers with a massive body build, thereby ensuring that a high proportion of the total mass propelled represents active muscle mass rather than the "dead-weight" of the cox and the vessel. Accordingly, the body mass of rowers should represent a high proportion of muscle (Fig. 3.1). For example, muscle mass in national level male open class rowers is around 59 kg, which corresponded to 62% of the whole body mass. Equally, the 168 male junior competitors at the 1997 World Junior Rowing Championships had a muscle mass of 50.2 kg corresponding to 62.4% of whole body mass. A similar percentage of muscle mass is demonstrated in lightweight rowers (58% of the whole body mass), while the total muscle mass is lower (42.6 kg). These data demonstrate that the proportion of muscle mass to the whole body mass does not change much from juniors to adult rowers, suggesting that the differences in performance result from talent and training rather than the equal relative muscle mass. As rowing is an endurance sport, approximately 60% of the muscle mass may be optimal. Approximately 75% of the total muscle mass (about 44 kg or 46% of the total body mass) is used in rowing. However, a large muscle mass does not penalize rowers, because their body mass is supported in the boat while in most other endurance disciplines high body mass is a limiting factor. Furthermore, a relationship

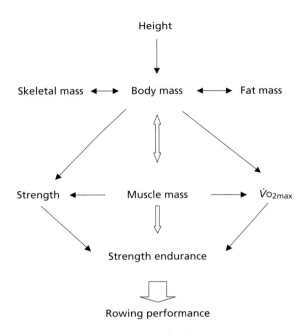

Fig. 3.1 Relationships between body mass components and rowing performance. $\dot{V}O_{2max}$, maximal oxygen consumption.

between muscle mass and 2000 m rowing performance time on rowing ergometer and on single sculls is established.

Perhaps because it is difficult to combine muscularity with leanness, a number of crews also carry a substantial amount of body fat. For example, a mean body fat percentage over 15% and 25% in elite open class male and female rowers, respectively, has been found, although it has decreased in recent years. In Olympic competitors, a mean of 8% in men and 15% for women has been measured. The mean body fat of the participants of the 1997 World Junior Rowing Championships was 11.3% and 22.8% for boys and girls, respectively, with no significant differences between sculling and sweep rowers. In elite open class rowers, there appears to be no change in body composition parameters between in-season and off-season, while lightweight rowers reduce their body fat mass without changing their fat-free mass. Typically, lightweight rowers reduce their body mass by 3–4% in the days before a competition. The level of adiposity in lightweight rowers is typically lower than untrained individuals. Male World Championship medalists have less

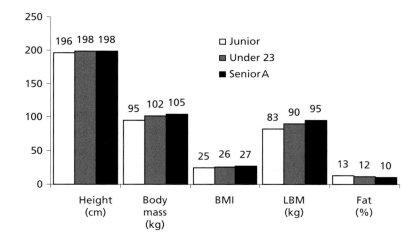

Fig. 3.2 Development of anthropometric parameters of the elite rower from junior to senior A level. BMI, body mass index; LBM, lean body mass.

adipose tissue and greater muscle mass than less successful athletes. The average body mass of male rowers increases about 15 kg until the end of growth at the age 19 of which ~85% represents muscle mass.

Figure 3.2 shows the body composition requirements for an elite male rower, who has been successful in World Championships regattas starting from junior age to the Senior A level. The height of the rower shows almost no change, while at the same time the weight increases. As body mass index does not change and body fat percentage decreases somewhat, the weight gain is accomplished with the increase in lean body mass, which mainly characterizes increases in muscle mass.

In conclusion, there are no large differences in height between junior and open class rowers, while open class rowers are heavier. Accordingly, specific body composition requirements and continuous adaptation are prerequisites for competitive success in different age categories and a carefully designed training plan for increasing muscle mass, while maintaining aerobic capacity, remains important.

Skeletal muscle characteristics

The muscles of highly trained rowers are able to develop force and power at relatively low contraction velocities. Muscular forces generated during competitive rowing are much higher when compared with other endurance sport disciplines. However, force must be maintained for more than

200 strokes during the 2000 m distance. In elite male rowers, the power that is applied to the boat averages about 420 W, which is approximately 70% of the highest power obtained during five maximal strokes in elite rowers. This observation demonstrates that the working muscles of rowers should possess relative high strength characteristics to produce sufficient force and also relative endurance characteristics to maintain the produced force. However, maximal strength of rowers is not correlated with rowing performance.

Skeletal muscle consists of different fibers and the strength of the single muscle fiber is a function of its cross-sectional area. Skeletal muscle possesses two main types of fibers, slow (ST) and fast twitch (FT). ST fibers have relatively slow contractile speed, high oxidative but low glycolytic capacity and high degree of fatigue resistance, making them suitable for endurance activities. FT fibers possess a relatively fast contractile speed, a low oxidative but high glycolytic capacity and they fatigue more quickly than ST fibers. However, FT fibers contract more quickly than ST fibers and may produce a greater force. FT fibers can be divided into FTa (fast twitch oxidative-glycolytic) and FTx (fast twitch glycolytic) fibers, the latter contracting extremely fast but having little resistance to fatigue. FTx fibers produce energy extremely quickly and have very low percentage of aerobic energy supply, so they are suitable for sprinting activities. The contractile speed of different muscle fiber types is determined by the myosin molecules and ST, FTa and FTx muscle fibers present

pH 4.37

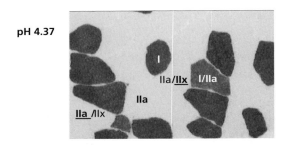

pH 4.60

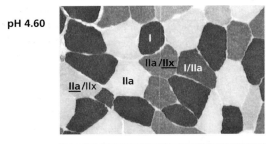

pH 10.30

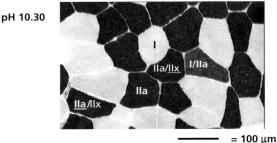

━━━━━ = 100 μm

Fig. 3.3 Cross-sectional view of a skeletal muscle with identification of three muscle fiber types (I, slow twitch fibers; IIa, fast twitch trained fibers; IIx, fast twitch untrained fibers) by ATPase staining after incubation at pH as indicated. (Jesper Løvig Andersen, Copenhagen Muscle Research Center.)

Table 3.3 Muscle fiber characteristics in different muscles of male rowers (Steinacker 1993).

Studied rowers	ST fibers	FTa fibers	FTx fibers
Performers ($n = 24$)	76.2 ± 5.8	3.8 ± 0.7	20.0 ± 5.7
Non-performers ($n = 28$)	66.1 ± 9.5	11.8 ± 3.0	22.1 ± 6.0
Stroke ($n = 34$)	67.7 ± 9.2	8.9 ± 5.4	23.4 ± 5.4
Bow ($n = 31$)	74.4 ± 10.2	7.9 ± 5.5	17.7 ± 5.5

FTa, fast twitch oxydative-glycolytic fibers; FTx, fast twitch glycolytic fibers; ST, slow twitch muscle fibers.

International level rowers have a percentage of enlarged ST fibers as high as 85%, with the remainder of the fibers being mostly FTa, which allow them to perform at submaximal intensities with lower lactate levels and thus are more economical compared with rowers with a high percentage of FT fibers. Furthermore, maximal lactate values are lower in rowers with a high percentage of ST fibers. Successful rowers present more FTa fibers at the expense of FTx fibers compared with non-athletes.

The muscle fiber type characteristics are also specific to the rower's position in the boat. A greater percentage of FT fibers has been found in stroke than in bow rowers. This may be because stroke rowers need to have a very quick catch. In all rowers, however, both FT and ST fibers present substantial hypertrophy in the main muscles that contribute to the rowing stroke and the degree of hypertrophy is not related to the position in the boat. The hypertrophy of ST fibers is more pronounced in internationally successful rowers. It can be suggested that the intense endurance training over several years in elite rowers causes the conversion of faster muscle fibers into slower ones (i.e., FTx → FTa and maybe even ST) so that working muscles are more fatigue resistant. Such training adaptation is brought about by the synthesis of slower myosin molecules resulting in hybrid fibers containing more than one type of myosin molecule.

The capillary to muscle fiber ratio is high in successful rowers as the number of capillaries increases with fiber area. Such athletes also demonstrate high oxidative metabolic capacity, elevated levels of succinate dehydrogenase and citrate synthase indicative of many and large mitochondria.

mainly, but not solely, type I, IIa and IIx myosin heavy chain isoforms, respectively (Fig. 3.3).

Most skeletal muscles contain all three muscle fiber types, the proportion depending on specific muscles. In rowing, primarily two muscle fiber types, ST and FTa, are important (Table 3.3). Successful rowers have more ST fibers in working muscles compared with less successful rowers, although their training time and volume is similar. Specifically, successful rowers are characterized by about 70% ST fibers in the quadriceps femoris muscle compared with about 50% in non-athletes.

In contrast, the glycolytic enzymes are not unusually developed, although better rowers demonstrate high percentages of the lactate dehydrogenase subtypes 1–3. In addition, the elevated absolute number of mitochondria, expressed as the ratio of mitochondria to fiber area, is evident in both ST and FT fibers.

Conclusions

• Large body mass and body size are performance related characteristics in rowing
• Differences in anthropometric parameters of rowers can be found between weight categories, boat classes, and among successful and less successful athletes
• Relatively high muscle mass is found in rowers compared to other endurance sports
• Successful rowers are characterized by a very high amount (>85%) of slow twitch muscle fibers
• Training-induced changes to the conversion of fast muscle fibers to slower muscle fibers may take place in successful rowers

References

Bourgois, J., Claessens, A.L. & Vrijens, J. (1998) *Hazewinkel Athropometric Project 1997. A study of world class male and female junior rowers*. Vlaamse Trainerschool, BLOSO, Brüssels.

Hagerman, F.C. (2000) The physiology of competitive rowing. In: W. Garrett Jr. & D.T. Kirkendall, eds. *Exercise and Sport Science*. Lippincott Williams & Wilkins, Philadelphia. pp. 843–873.

Steinacker, J.M. (1993) Physiological aspects of rowing. *International Journal of Sports Medicine* **14**, 3–10.

Recommended reading

Claessens, A.L., Bourgois, J., Beunen, G., *et al.* (2003) Age at menarche in relation to anthropometric characteristics, competition level and boat category in elite junior rowers. *Annals of Human Biology* **30**, 148–159.

Mäestu J., Jürimäe J. & Jürimäe T. (2005) Monitoring of performance and training in rowing. *Sports Medicine* **35**, 597–617.

Shephard, R.J. (1998) Science and medicine of rowing: A review. *Sports Science* **16**, 603–620.

Chapter 4
Physiology

N.H. Secher, S. Volianitis and J. Jürimäe

Metabolic cost

The metabolic cost of rowing reflects mainly the power used to overcome the drag force of the boat in the water. Hence, it would be expected that, according to fluid dynamics (Chapter 2), as the power required for propulsion increases with speed approximately to the third power, the metabolic cost would increase accordingly. However, measurements of oxygen uptake ($\dot{V}O_2$) while rowing a single scull, a double scull and a pair, have shown that the metabolic cost of rowing increases with speed only to the 2.4 power (Fig. 4.1).

Such determinations are confounded by the fact that the $\dot{V}O_2$ value represents not only the metabolic cost of the boat's propulsion, but also that of the body's backward and forward movements. The relationship between $\dot{V}O_2$ and "unloaded" rowing at different rowing frequencies is linear and it should be considered that this component of $\dot{V}O_2$ may be as much as $4 \, L \cdot min^{-1}$. If the $\dot{V}O_2$ component of the "unloaded" rowing is subtracted from the determined $\dot{V}O_2$, then the $\dot{V}O_2$ used for propulsion increases with speed to the 3.1 power. However, because the movement of the body during the recovery part of the stroke contributes to the propulsion of the boat, up to half of the "unloaded" rowing $\dot{V}O_2$ may also have a role in the propulsion of the boat.

Depending on the boat type, a 2000 m race may require between 220 and 250 strokes to complete, with the forces being exerted on the oar handle for each stroke being the equivalent of 400–500 N. As a consequence, rowers require very high muscular strength and power in order to sustain maximal effort during a race, which typically lasts 5.5–7.5 min (see Table 1.5). The mechanical efficiency of rowing at less than 25 strokes·min⁻¹ is 18% and it increases to 20–23% at 35 strokes·min⁻¹. Hence, the metabolic cost of a race calculated from actual rowing times and assuming a constant mechanical efficiency of 22%, ranges 6.7–$7.0 \, L \, O_2 \cdot min^{-1}$ for men, $5.9 \, L \, O_2 \cdot min^{-1}$ for lightweight men, $5.3 \, L \, O_2 \cdot min^{-1}$ for women and $4.9 \, L \, O_2 \cdot min^{-1}$ for lightweight women, and these values increase by approximately 200 mL per decade. Even though the most valid method of physiologic testing is to measure $\dot{V}O_2$ on the water, using a Douglas bag or a telemetric $\dot{V}O_2$ monitor, a six-minute "all-out" and, more recently, a 2000 m ergometer effort have been used as a simulation of a rowing competition. A kinematic comparison of rowing and rowing ergometry shows that the dominant movements of the legs and trunk are similar for the two types of activity and ergometry yields very similar aerobic power values to those obtained on the water.

Energy requirements and cardiorespiratory limitations

There are many different physiologic and anthropometric parameters that can be used alone or in combination with other parameters to predict the competitive success of rowers. However, it appears that one of the most important physiologic determinants of rowing performance is absolute maximal oxygen consumption ($\dot{V}O_{2max}$ L·min⁻¹). During the classic 2000 m rowing competition, rowers depend mainly on their aerobic metabolism because of limited glycolytic energy stores. On average, about 75–80% of the energy comes from aerobic energy systems and the remaining 20–25% from anaerobic energy systems. Therefore, obtaining high aerobic power values is of much importance for a successful rower, and the training of rowers is also characterized by large amounts of low intensity training under the 4 mmol lactate threshold. Anaerobic energy systems are used mainly during the start phase of the race (for approximately 60–80 s)

because of the very high power required to overcome the inertia of the boat and to set to the race pace, while it takes a minute or so for oxygen uptake to reach its maximal level (Fig. 4.2).

Anaerobic energy is produced in lesser amounts also during the finish of the race. Aerobic power can be defined as the maximal oxygen consumption which describes the highest amount of oxygen that a body can utilize during heavy strenuous exercise. This value integrates the ability of the lungs to provide oxygen to blood, the oxygen binding capacities of the blood, maximum cardiac output, type of muscles and the amount of capillaries surrounding the muscle. The schematic view of the main organ systems that are involved in the development of high $\dot{V}O_{2max}$ and their trainability is presented in Fig. 4.3. Even though limitations to rowing performance vary depending on the duration of the event and ambient temperature, oxygen transport from the atmosphere to the working muscles remains critical. During rowing no single factor limits the oxygen transport cascade expressed as the sum of the resistances presented by each step. Yet, in order to preserve arterial pressure, blood flow to working muscles and internal organs, including the brain, is restrained with adverse outcomes for metabolism and fatigue. In this chapter, oxygen transport in the body is followed with little address to inter-individual differences in oxygen-carrying capacity.

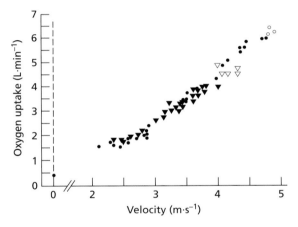

Fig. 4.1 $\dot{V}O_2$ of two oarsmen during rowing a single scull. The regression equation is $\dot{V}O_2 = 0.1944\,v^{2.21} + 0.28$, the resting metabolic rate.

Aerobic metabolism

Over the course of a 2000 m race, elite rowers exercise at a "severe steady state," with the majority of

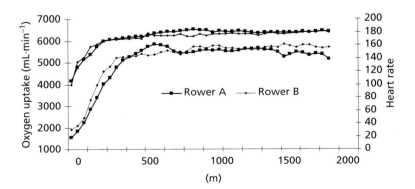

Fig. 4.2 Oxygen consumption ($\dot{V}O_{2max}$) and heart rate values during a 2000 m simulated rowing race in two rowers.

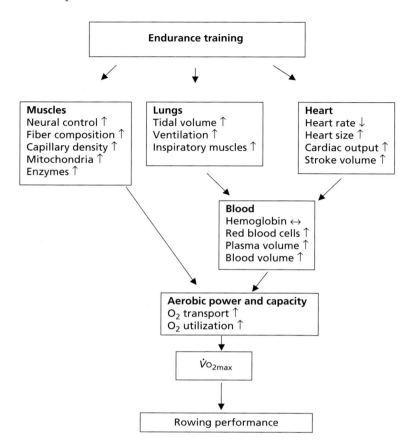

Fig. 4.3 Organ systems and their trainability to impact maximal oxygen consumption ($\dot{V}O_{2max}$) and rowing performance.

Table 4.1 Anthropometric and physiologic data of rowers compared with sedentary people.

Category	Height (cm)	Weight (kg)	$\dot{V}O_{2max}$ (L·min^{-1})	$\dot{V}_E$ (L·min^{-1})	SV (mL)	CO (L·min^{-1})
Sedentary female	168	65	2.5	100	71	15
Sedentary male	178	75	3.3	135	100	20
Junior female	177	72	4.0	150	145	28
Junior male	190	85	5.1	170	160	31
Lightweight female	170	57	4.0	150	145	31
Lightweight male	184	70	5.1	170	160	35
Elite female	182	80	4.5	170	180	35
Elite male	195	95	6.5	>200	200	40

CO, cardiac output; SV, heart stroke volume; $\dot{V}_E$, minute ventilation; $\dot{V}O_{2max}$, maximal oxygen consumption.

work performed between 95% and 98% of maximal aerobic capacity. Male national and elite level heavyweight rowers have a $\dot{V}O_2$ of up to 6 L·min^{-1} and 6.5 L·min^{-1}, respectively, while heavyweight female rowers have about 4 and 4.4 L·min^{-1}, respectively (Table 4.1). Lightweight men have a $\dot{V}O_2$ of up to 5.6 L·min^{-1} while their female counterparts have 4 L·min^{-1}. There has been a strong linear relationship ($r = 0.99$) established between placement in a Fédération Internationale des Sociétés d'Aviron

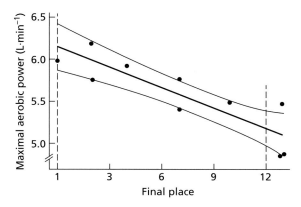

Fig. 4.4 Regression line between average $\dot{V}O_{2max}$ of a crew and placement in the 1971 FISA championship. The 95% confidence limits of the regression are also shown.

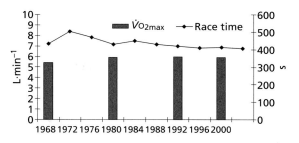

Fig. 4.5 Changes in average maximal oxygen consumption ($\dot{V}O_{2max}$) in male international rowers over the last 30 year period.

(FISA) championship and the crew's average $\dot{V}O_{2max}$ (Fig. 4.4).

The racing pattern commonly used in a 2000 m rowing race is unique. This is depicted by a short sprint of about 40 s at the start, requiring a large energy turnover, placing large demands on the anaerobic energy system, and a high cadence of about 40–50 strokes·min^{-1}. During the middle part of the race the stroke rate is reduced and maintained at 34–38 strokes·min^{-1} before increasing again over the last minute of the race. A physiologic explanation for the initial spurt performed is the linear relationship between the rate of oxygen uptake increase at the onset of exercise and the work output. Accordingly, the total oxygen uptake and work output during a given period of exercise is larger when an initial spurt is performed than when one attempts to keep exercise at an average intensity throughout a race. Oxygen uptake reaches its highest value after 90 s and balances out at a level that shows only a slight decrease during the remaining 4 min. The $\dot{V}O_{2max}$ of rowers has increased over the years by approximately 3.4 L·min^{-1}; however, the average $\dot{V}O_{2max}$ has not changed much during the last 20 years in international level rowers while at the same time racing times for single sculls for male rowers continues to decrease (Fig. 4.5).

Seasonal changes in $\dot{V}O_{2max}$ have been described with increases of 5–15 mL·min^{-1}·kg^{-1} or ~10% during the competitive season. However, increases in relative values of $\dot{V}O_{2max}$ may be highly dependent on

decreases in body mass which can also be observed in national level rowers, while almost no change is found among elite rowers. An increase in $\dot{V}O_{2max}$ from 5.1 to 6.0 L·min^{-1}, from off-season to in-season, among USA Olympic rowers has been observed. However, different studies have also demonstrated no substantial changes in $\dot{V}O_{2max}$ over the season in elite athletes. Pronounced decreases in the $\dot{V}O_{2max}$ of highly trained rowers can take place during off-season if the distance rowed is reduced below approximately 100 km·week^{-1}.

$\dot{V}O_{2max}$ is an important predictor of competitive success, as indicated by the relationship between $\dot{V}O_{2max}$ and on-water rowing performance in several studies. $\dot{V}O_{2max}$ increases with age, training distance per year and with rowing experience. Usually, $\dot{V}O_{2max}$ levels off at about the age of 18 but increases can be seen as a consequence of endurance training until the beginning of Senior A level (i.e., the age of 24) (Fig. 4.6). In parallel, increases can be seen in other endurance parameters.

A plateau in $\dot{V}O_{2max}$ has been observed in highly trained rowers despite increased training volumes. Even with the attainment of a plateau in $\dot{V}O_{2max}$, rowers can still improve their performance. This can be achieved by increasing the endurance capacity — the ability of maintaining higher $\dot{V}O_2$ during the distance (up to 98% of $\dot{V}O_{2max}$) manifested as high average power during the race. Because endurance capacity appears to be important in performance prediction when rowers of similar $\dot{V}O_{2max}$ values are compared and the correlation between $\dot{V}O_{2max}$ and performance may be rather poor, alternative parameters for the measurement of endurance capacity have been proposed. For example, it is

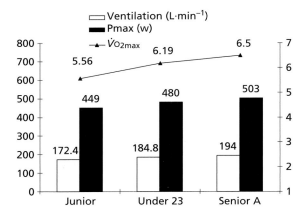

Fig. 4.6 The development of maximal oxygen consumption ($\dot{V}O_{2max}$), ventilation and maximal aerobic power (P_{max}) of elite rowers from junior to Senior A level.

suggested that the submaximal endurance capacity measured at the power that elicits a blood lactate level of 4.0 mmol·L^{-1} is the most predictive parameter for competition performance in trained rowers, especially in smaller boats such as singles and doubles. Rowers with high $\dot{V}O_2$ values at the intensity that elicits a blood lactate concentration of 4.0 mmol·L^{-1} perform better in 6–7 min maximal tests than rowers with lower values of $\dot{V}O_2$ at the same level of blood lactate concentration. During the simulated 2000 m rowing race, the $\dot{V}O_2$ can also be measured. The advantage of this testing instead of the "classic" incremental test is that it allows the measurement of the average $\dot{V}O_2$ uptake during the distance. However, during this testing, where usually maximal values occur within the first 2 min, $\dot{V}O_{2max}$ may be higher than during the graded exercise test.

The difference between $\dot{V}O_{2max}$ values achieved in different tests is probably a function of task specificity. Moreover, during incremental testing, the athletes reach maximum intensities at about 15 min after the start of the test. This may cause slightly higher strain on the cardiovascular system and skeletal muscles and therefore lower $\dot{V}O_{2max}$ values. Figure 4.2 represents the $\dot{V}O_2$ data for two male rowers during a simulated 2000 m rowing ergometer race. The $\dot{V}O_{2max}$ for rower A was 6.10 L·min^{-1} and for rower B was 5.87 L·min^{-1} during the graded exercise test. However, despite significant difference between $\dot{V}O_{2max}$ values, their 2000 m performance

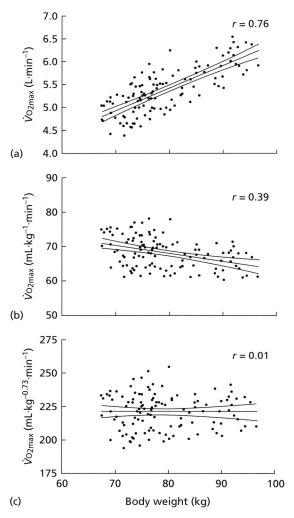

Fig. 4.7 Relationship between $\dot{V}O_{2max}$ and body mass for 117 male rowers. Regression lines with 95% confidence intervals and correlation coefficients (r) are shown. (a) The $\dot{V}O_{2max}$ increases with body mass, but when it is expressed relative to body mass (b), those subjects with the largest body mass show the smallest values, even when trained for the same sport. (c) When scaling $\dot{V}O_{2max}$ with body mass to the 0.73 power (i.e., mL·kg$^{-0.73}$·min^{-1}), $\dot{V}O_{2max}$ becomes independent of body mass. (Jensen *et al.* 2001.)

difference was only 2 s. Furthermore, their $\dot{V}O_{2max}$ during the 2000 m tests were almost equal, 5.84 and 5.83 L·min^{-1}, respectively. These data elucidate the importance of the testing method on $\dot{V}O_{2max}$ values for performance predictions.

Finally, body size is a determinant of $\dot{V}O_{2max}$, with a 0.73 power association to body weight (Fig. 4.7), illustrating an advantage for light persons when the body weight is lifted as during running, as opposed to when the body weight is supported as during rowing which favors large heavy individuals.

Anaerobic metabolism

Anaerobic metabolism is indicated by a high peak blood lactate concentration, which increases with the muscle mass involved in exercise and the motivation of the rowers. Values of 11 mmol·L^{-1} have been reported after treadmill running, 15 mmol·L^{-1} after a national regatta, and 17 mmol·L^{-1} following a FISA championship. Accordingly, the buffering system of the blood (bicarbonate) decreases from 26 to 13 mmol·L^{-1} after all-out rowing, and bicarbonate may in fact be eliminated from the blood. This means that the pH of the blood decreases from its normal value of 7.4 to 7.1 after all-out rowing. The record low pH value of 6.74, corresponding to a blood lactate level of 32 mmol·L^{-1}, was measured following a championship ergometer rowing where bicarbonate was completely depleted and the highest blood lactate level measured was 36 mmol·L^{-1} in a World Champion rower.

However, these values give little indication of the amount of anaerobic metabolism. For that purpose the "oxygen deficit," which is the part of metabolism that is not covered by $\dot{V}O_2$ uptake during exercise, can be calculated. In rowers, the oxygen deficit has been reported to be 88–97 mL·kg^{-1}, or substantially larger than that reported in runners. However, the anaerobic contribution to metabolism has not been determined for the duration of races, and even for 6-min all-out ergometer rowing, estimates vary between 21% and 30%.

Endocrine and metabolic responses

In response to mental and physical stress, circulating eosinophils decrease from 108 to 19 mm^{-3} before a race, and even to 3 mm^{-3} after exhaustive rowing, while adenocorticotropic hormone (ACTH) and adrenaline increase. After ergometer rowing, plasma epinephrine and norepinephrine concentrations increase from resting values of 0.9 and 2.3 nmol·L^{-1}, respectively, to extremely high values

of 19 and 74 nmol·L^{-1}. These values are about twice as large as those noted during running, suggesting a role for muscle mass in the catecholamine response to maximal exercise. Also, pancreatic polypeptide, a hormone under vagal control, increases from 21 to 48 pmol·L^{-1} after ergometer rowing, suggesting that vagal activity may contribute to the feeling of fatigue including gastrointestinal symptoms experienced at exhaustion.

Protein turnover is greater in oarsmen than in controls but the calculated protein synthesis is not increased in oarsmen, supporting the view that intense exercise does not increase basal protein turnover rate in adequately nourished individuals. Serum androgen and growth hormone increase from 690 ng·mL^{-1} and 5 μU·mL^{-1}, respectively, at rest to 840 ng·mL^{-1} and 49 μU·mL^{-1} after maximal running, but do not increase after submaximal rowing. These changes occur despite a constant serum luteinizing hormone (62 ng·mL^{-1}). It may be speculated that the raised level of androgen during exercise acts in association with growth hormone to increase the pubertal growth velocity and contributes to muscular development associated with exercise. Administration of testosterone, however, does not increase muscle glycogen build-up after maximal dynamic exercise. Serum concentration of myoglobin and creatinine kinase (a cellular enzyme) are elevated after 10 km rowing and remain elevated 1.5 h after the training bout, indicating skeletal muscle cellular damage which could help explain muscle soreness after rowing.

Ventilation

The lung is the organ for exchange of gases between air and blood. Carbon dioxide produced from metabolism is unloaded to the alveoli while O_2 diffuses into the blood in the opposite direction where it binds to hemoglobin. The transport is solely passive and the driving force is based on the gas pressure gradients between blood and air. Until the beginning of the 20th century, the fundamental idea was that O_2 was actively secreted by lung cells. The consideration that O_2 transport may be limited by diffusion in the lungs was first recognized some

30 years ago. Thus, it is questioned whether the lung is "built for exercise" and in particular for rowing.

At rest, ventilation involves activation of the diaphragm muscle, which operates as a motor piston to generate a negative pressure within the thorax whereby external air passively enters the lung alveoli. During exercise, the diaphragm operates with increased force while the external respiratory muscles help to expand the ribcage and further decrease the intrathoracic pressure. Thus, increased minute ventilation ($\dot{V}_E$) is generated by increased breathing frequency and increased depth of each breath. Very large respiratory minute volumes are developed during rowing competition, typically greater than $200\,L\cdot min^{-1}$ and sometimes as high as $250\text{--}270\,L\cdot min^{-1}$. During the 6 min all-out rowing, $\dot{V}_E$ rises exponentially until the third minute when the rate of increase slows down, but nevertheless, it continuous to increase until the end of the effort. Even though rowers assume a cramped body position during the initial phase of the stroke, which presumably could impair normal excursion of the diaphragm, the ventilation to oxygen uptake ratio ($\dot{V}_E : \dot{V}_{O_2}$) equals or exceeds that of most other endurance athletes. The ventilatory volumes observed during maximal rowing are the highest reported in competitive sports. It could be argued that, because breathing frequency does not differ between trained and untrained, the lung is built for rowing, as performance capacity is more favorable for rowers with large total lung and vital capacities (VC). Hence, the lungs of rowers reflect their large bodies, and a VC up to 9.1 L has been recorded. This observation may, however, be reflecting natural selection as total lung capacity or VC is the only link of the oxygen transport chain that does not improve with training once adult stature has been attained and even decreases with age. Thus, a correlation between rowing performance and VC is reported regularly and rowers typically demonstrate VC values of 7 L compared to 5.5 L as expected for their body size.

On the other hand, the largest ventilatory volume could be considered to be a disadvantage as a large ventilation requires a higher activation of ventilatory muscles which appear to compete for their share of cardiac output. In fact, unloading of breathing by mechanical assistance increases blood flow to skeletal muscles and specific training of the inspiratory (but not the expiratory) muscles is reported to enhance rowing performance.

Breathing pattern

During rowing, breathing is entrained to the rowing stroke meaning that expiration and inspiration are performed in phase with the rowing stroke. The $\dot{V}_E$ and the pattern of breathing during rowing are the result of respiratory muscle contraction acting on the mechanical properties of the respiratory system. The tidal volume is determined by the size of the lungs, and both inspiratory and expiratory times are influenced by maximum airflow. Maximal tidal volume during simulated competitive rowing averages ~55% of VC. Inspiratory flow rate is limited primarily by the ability to generate inspiratory muscle pressure, while expiratory flow rate is limited by airway mechanics, not the ability to generate expiratory pressure. Peak expiratory flow rates reach values of $15\,L\cdot s^{-1}$ in elite male rowers, but some of these individuals also show a plateau in expiratory flow rates suggestive of airway collapse.

Female rowers have higher specific static and dynamic lung compliance and lower recoil pressure at functional residual capacity compared with other female athletes or male rowers. The physical stress on the thorax during rowing is not comparable between women and men, because of the extra trunk length of about 2 cm located in the abdominal region for reproductive purposes. Hence, in contrast to men, women require additional static muscular work to stabilize their relatively longer trunk during the drive phase of the stroke. This stabilizing action is manifested with fixation of the diaphragm and the abdominal muscles and is reflected in measurements of transpulmonary pressure during rowing where the intrathoracic pressure rises during the drive phase in female but not in male rowers.

The reduced lung elastance is responsible for the significant expiratory flow limitation observed in female and, to a lesser degree, in male rowers. As a result, a dynamic hyperinflation of the lungs with concomitant functional consequences develops. These consequences are: (i) increased elastic work; (ii) reduced mechanical efficiency of the respiratory muscles as a result of a suboptimal length–tension relationship; and (iii) by combining the two previous points, increased predisposition to respiratory muscle fatigue and dyspnea.

Entrainment, or synchronization between limb movements and breathing pattern, is a common occurrence during rowing and, although the exact "stimulus" remains unclear, several factors are associated with it. Because contraction of the thoracic musculature is required both for respiration and stabilization of the trunk during rowing, it is important that breathing and rowing stroke are synchronized so that one does not interfere with the other. The physiologic benefits from such coupling are most likely an improvement in the efficiency of the respiratory muscles and gas exchange, prevention of diaphragmatic fatigue, and reduction of breathing effort sensation. Hence, the rowing movement influences the respiratory efficiency and, at the same time, respiratory muscles modulate the rowing stroke.

Even though it seems that the cramped body position assumed by the rower at the start of the rowing stroke would impair diaphragmatic excursions and modify the adopted breathing pattern, nevertheless, greater diaphragmatic limitation exists at the finish position than at the catch. This limitation is attributed to the transient abdominal pressure induced by the co-contraction of the diaphragm and the abdominal muscles at the finish to stabilize the upper body. Expiring during the drive phase creates a higher intra-abdominal pressure at the mid-drive position that partially compensates for the high shear and compression forces that the lower lumbar vertebrae are exposed to. A structural manifestation of what is essentially a Valsalva maneuver is the cardiac hypertrophy found in rowers.

During incremental rowing ergometry ventilatory tidal volume progressively increases up to the point where each breath encroaches upon the flat portion of the pulmonary compliance curve. Hence, a greater portion of the negative intrapleural pressure is used to overcome pulmonary elastic work. To circumvent this mechanical limitation of lung distension during inspiration, rowers shift from a 1:1 to a 2:1 breath:stroke ratio. The respiratory system is then confronted with a different mechanical constraint, that of expiratory flow limitation, because of the limited time of each expiratory phase.

During a simulated 2000 m race, rowers breathe at similar times in the stroke cycle at a 2:1 breath:stroke ratio. Inspiration occurs most frequently during the first 40% of the recovery phase, followed by expiration during the latter part of this phase. The above-mentioned breathing pattern also explains how high breathing frequency (60–90 times per minute) can be reached by elite rowers. It seems that there are advantageous times in the stroke for large inspired and expired volumes and breaths are taken at times where muscle synergy produces larger volumes for a given amount of respiratory work or, alternatively, the same volume for less respiratory work.

Diffusion capacity

Oxygen enters the body through the lungs which have an enormous gas diffusion capacity with an alveolar area of 50–100 m^2. Increased ventilation is coupled intimately to exercise but during submaximal and maximal rowing, the contribution of the lungs to oxygen transport remains unknown for two reasons. Lung function is described as a capacity rather than as the actual contribution to transport of oxygen during rowing. Furthermore, evaluation of the lungs is combined with the capacity of hemoglobin in pulmonary capillaries to take up oxygen, expressed as the *pulmonary diffusion capacity* (DLCO) using carbon monoxide (CO) as test gas. The more relevant value of diffusion capacity for oxygen is 23% larger than DLCO and the value for carbon dioxide is 24.6 times DLCO.

DLCO is a non-invasive measure of lung function using CO as test gas because its affinity to hemoglobin is 200 times that of oxygen. When ~1% CO is added to inspired air, CO is binding with hemoglobin over the entire length of the pulmonary capillary (Fig. 4.8) and under these conditions DLCO represents the gas transport capacity.

Conversely, DLCO is dominated by acute changes of the pulmonary capillary blood volume. For example, DLCO decreases by 15% from the supine to the seated position at rest because pulmonary capillary blood volume is reduced while the pulmonary membrane diffusion is enhanced by 30%.

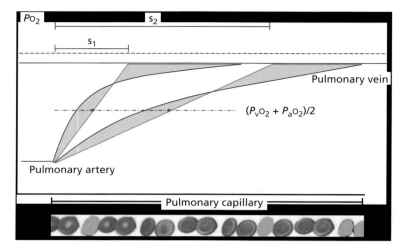

Fig. 4.8 Diagram of oxygen tension of blood (PO_2) during its course through a pulmonary capillary at two flow rates. Also shown a cartoon of red cells passing a pulmonary capillary with carbon monoxide (CO) binding to hemoglobin. The apparent pulmonary diffusion for oxygen (DmO_2) expresses the effective area for diffusion rather than the diffusion capacity established when the whole capillary is engaged in oxygen transfer. Because there is little or no transport of oxygen in the venous end of the capillary, the effective capillary diffusion area (s_1 or s_2) is approximated by the insertion of a line integrating the considered increase in PO_2. When it takes longer for the alveolar to capillary oxygen equilibrium to be established because of doubled flow during exercise or because of low inspired oxygen tension, the venous end of the capillary becomes increasingly important and an enhanced effective diffusion area is expressed as an elevated DmO_2. Discrepancy between a doubling of the diffusion capacity for CO and a eightfold increase in DmO_2 during exercise indicates that at rest in normoxia, an equilibrium is established between PAO_2 and PCO_2 within one-quarter of the length of the pulmonary capillary. During hypoxemia, however, an equilibrium is not reached and the entire capillary contributes to diffusion expressed as a maximal DmO_2. Any venous admixture to arterial blood is reported as a change in DmO_2 representing an integrated measure of pulmonary function rather than of diffusion per se. To validate the absolute value pulmonary venous oxygen tension needs to replace PaO_2 in the calculation of DmO_2.

During rowing, there is a doubling of DLCO (25–50 mL·mmHg^{-1}·min^{-1}), reflecting a support of the muscle pump to the pulmonary capillaries blood volume with recruitment of pulmonary capillaries in the apical parts of the lungs (Fig. 4.9).

Transport of oxygen

In contrast to CO taken up over the entire length of the capillary, in normoxia equilibrium between alveolar and capillary oxygen tensions is established within a fraction of the capillary blood transit time (Fig. 4.8). During rowing, as the velocity of red cells in pulmonary capillaries increases, equilibrium takes longer to be established and, ultimately, as the length of the capillary is involved in the diffusion of oxygen, the diffusion capacity is utilized.

As the length of the capillary involved in diffusion increases during rowing, it becomes difficult to maintain alveolar oxygen tension (PAO_2) and an increase in ventilation is required to compensate for oxygen taken up by capillary blood. During rowing, ventilation follows two distinct patterns. Low intensity rowing is associated with little drive to ventilation representing the influence from the central nervous system (*central command*). Relative hypoventilation is expressed as a ~4 mmHg elevation of the arterial CO_2 tension ($PaCO_2$), which is the dominant stimulus for ventilation at rest. As workload progresses, ventilation increases exponentially influenced by the decreased blood pH. The important effect of blood pH on driving ventilation is demonstrated by the ~15 L·min^{-1} reduced ventilation following normalization of pH with bicarbonate administration despite the 7.5 mmHg increase

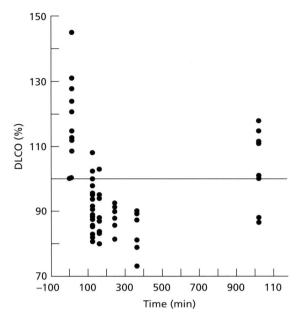

Fig. 4.9 Pulmonary diffusion capacity following 6 min all-out ergometer rowing. Courtesy of B. Hanel, Copenhagen Muscle Research Center.

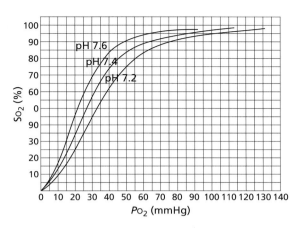

Fig. 4.10 The oxyhemoglobin dissociation curve.

of $PaCO_2$. During intense rowing, the marked hyperventilation decreases $PaCO_2$ below the resting value and PAO_2 increases to high levels (128 mmHg).

Even though during light to moderate rowing the lungs facilitate O_2 transport by recruiting alveoli and enhancing the within-capillary diffusion area, a diffusion capacity of ~80 mL·mmHg^{-1}·min^{-1} (an eightfold increase from rest) is insufficient to account for the often more than 15-fold increase in $\dot{V}O_2$ during maximal rowing. Further, during intense rowing, $\dot{V}O_2$ depends on a widening of the alveolar–capillary oxygen tension difference because gas diffusion is impeded by high pulmonary artery pressure that provokes accumulation of fluid in the alveolar–capillary space. Thus, arterial oxygen tension (PaO_2), expressed as a physiologic shunt or exercise-induced hypoxemia, decreases (e.g., from 90 to 75 mmHg) although PAO_2 increases during intense rowing.

During intense rowing, the elevated ventilation, as demonstrated by the extraordinary large ventilatory rates observed in trained rowers (up to 270 L·min^{-1}), increases PAO_2 and, consequently, PaO_2 is maintained at the highest possible level. Such mechanism may explain the enhanced rowing performance following specific respiratory muscle training that supports a large ventilation and PaO_2 as indicated by the elevated endtidal O_2 tension during exercise. In contrast, pulmonary diffusion capacity does not seem to respond to training and the large reported values for DLCO represent selection of gifted individuals with exceptionally large VC as is the case for competitive rowers with ~7 L. DLCO varies from 15 to 45 mL·mmHg^{-1}·min^{-1} and this range reflects differences in body size and central blood volume besides variation in pulmonary membrane diffusion capacity. Pulmonary membrane diffusion capacity is larger than DLCO because it does not include the resistance to diffusion of O_2 in plasma, or the binding of CO to hemoglobin, while values for rowers versus control subjects, or for a potential effect of training, are not established.

Hemoglobin

Oxygen is dissolved in blood and it also binds to hemoglobin, whereby the O_2 carrying capacity in blood is markedly increased. Dissolved O_2, described by the PaO_2 (normal value 100 mmHg) which, together with the acidity of the blood (normal blood pH is 7.43), determine the level of hemoglobin saturated with O_2 (normal value 97–99%). The transport of O_2 in blood by hemoglobin is described by the oxyhemoglobin dissociation curve (Fig. 4.10) reserving ~2% of the transport to O_2 dissolved in plasma during maximal rowing.

At rest and during moderate rowing, where PaO_2 value is ~100 mmHg, pH has little influence on the

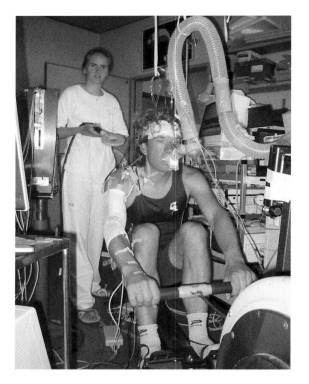

Fig. 4.11 Evaluation of ventilation and circulation during ergometer rowing.

amount of O_2 transported. During maximal rowing where, despite the increased drive to breath, PaO_2 is reduced to a level similar to that seen at rest in high altitude, a right-shift (Bohr effect) of the oxyhemoglobin dissociation curve demonstrates that any deviation in pH affects the ability of hemoglobin to transport oxygen and, consequently, $\dot{V}O_{2max}$ is affected in proportion to the reduction in hemoglobin saturation. During maximal ergometer rowing, the Bohr effect reduces arterial oxygen saturation to ~90% and imposes a 5–10% restrain on $\dot{V}O_{2max}$. In laboratory studies using oxygen-enriched air breathing, where the inspired O_2 fraction is increased from 0.21 to 0.30, PaO_2 is increased to above normal values and the influence of a low pH on hemoglobin O_2 binding is attenuated, resulting in the restoration of arterial O_2 saturation. Ventilation is not affected but with a higher O_2 pressure gradient and high O_2 hemoglobin saturation, blood O_2 carrying capacity increases, which appears to induce a higher O_2 uptake whereby rowing perform-

ance is enhanced by 2%. Arterial O_2 saturation is also restored in response to pH normalization, following bicarbonate administration, and $\dot{V}O_{2max}$ also increases (Fig. 4.11). On the other hand, O_2 delivery is enhanced both by the effect of rowing-induced body temperature elevation and the Bohr effect, augmented by the lower pH of venous compared to arterial blood (e.g., 7.0 vs. 7.2) as carbon dioxide is exhaled (PCO_2 reduced from 90 to 40 mmHg; venous vs. arterial).

The impact of the lung in limiting rowing performance is demonstrated as even a minute ventilation of more than 200 L is not enough to maintain the PaO_2 during maximal rowing and an even higher ventilation may offer some protection against the reduction in PaO_2. Therefore, in elite rowers ventilation does contribute to limit O_2 transport and it is also a factor that may discriminate winners and losers.

Blood lactate

The Bohr effect on the oxyhemoglobin dissociation curve illustrates the delicate balance between aerobic and anaerobic metabolism during maximal rowing, but little is known about that balance during actual competitions. Appreciating the various tactics rowers apply during a race, it is likely that the degree that oxygen transport is affected by acidity varies among individuals depending on PaO_2 which is influenced by the balance between hyperventilation and pulmonary membrane diffusion capacity. Rowing races start at high speed to accelerate the increase in $\dot{V}O_2$ because the total aerobic metabolism is represented by the accumulated oxygen uptake during the race rather than the highest level $\dot{V}O_2$ reaches.

More is known about rowing at high altitude. When the inspired oxygen tension is low, it is disadvantageous to work at an intensity that provokes lactate acidosis because any anaerobic contribution to metabolism attenuates the more important oxygen carrying capacity of blood. While it is possible to work at an intensity that provokes lactate acidosis, exercise in hypoxia is usually associated with a small deviation in pH, a condition that has been defined as the high altitude *lactate paradox*. Following high altitude acclimatization, where both ventilation and PaO_2 increase, plasma lactate during maximal rowing is comparable with the sea-level values. The unproven, but likely beneficial, effect of moderate altitude training (~2000 m) for sea-level performance may be explained by the adaptation of the respiratory muscles to the large rowing ventilation in hypoxia. Upon return to sea level, it feels easier to maintain high ventilation and elevate PaO_2 during competition, thus, enhance the anaerobic contribution to rowing without affecting the oxygen transport capacity of hemoglobin.

Lactate threshold

Interest has also focused on the lactate threshold or the work rate that elicits a blood lactate concentration of 4 mmol·L^{-1}. This work rate increases with training, and it seems to depend on the muscle fiber composition of the rower; those with many slow twitch fibers are able to exercise at a high intensity with a blood lactate value of no more than 4 mmol·L^{-1}.

The Bohr effect on the oxyhemoglobin dissociation curve explains why the work rate, at a given blood lactate level, is a sensitive predictor of rowing performance. Blood lactate increases exponentially with workload but their relationship is right-shifted following training (i.e., blood lactate increases with relative workload). The workload that elicits a given lactate level (often set at 4 mmol·L^{-1}) is, thereby, an indirect measure of $\dot{V}O_{2max}$ that, in itself, is a predictor of performance. Blood lactate is a more precise performance predictor because blood lactate reflects not only $\dot{V}O_{2max}$, but also the ability to work without affecting the oxyhemoglobin dissociation curve.

For a given workload less lactate is produced with the recruitment of ST rather than FT muscle fibers as illustrated when ST fibers are prevented from contracting with curare-induced (South American arrow poison) partial neuromuscular blockade. The workload that elicits a given blood lactate level reflects the work capacity of ST muscle fibers. The composition of muscles depends not only on the percentage of ST versus FT fibers, but also on their relative size. For example, weightlifters develop large FT fibers in adaptation to rapid lifts, while rowers are characterized by large ST fibers reflecting the relatively slow movements involved in rowing (see Fig. 3.3). Furthermore, considering that central fatigue inhibits ST muscle fiber recruitment, during rowing that requires increased central command, a smaller contribution to work from ST muscle fibers necessitates that work has to be carried out with a larger contribution from FT muscle fibers which results in elevated lactate production. In other words, evaluation of blood lactate during submaximal rowing reflects the mental preparation and automatization of the movement that determines the central command requirements.

Alongside these considerations it should also be noted that although it is lactate that is measured in blood, it is the deviation in pH that influences oxygen transport. Lactate is a substrate for tissues including muscle, liver, kidney and brain but its exponential accumulation in the blood as the work rate increases is a manifestation of attenuated elimination by liver and kidneys. Blood lactate is, thereby, also an indicator of how well organ blood flow is preserved during various rowing intensities.

The heart rate response

The heart rate response to rowing is of particular interest because the almost linear relationship between heart rate and workload (or $\dot{V}O_2$) is applied widely for evaluation of $\dot{V}O_{2max}$ in population studies. Furthermore, heart rate is also a determinant of cardiac output that supports blood pressure, which in turn affects perfusion of the working muscles and the brain. Hence, a brief presentation of the factors that affect heart rate, cardiac output, blood pressure and blood flow to vascular beds critical for rowing performance follows.

Blood volume and cardiac preload

The heart of quadrupedal animals is at a level with the main portion of blood within the body, but upright humans face a circulatory challenge as the indifference point for volume is at the level of the pelvis and about 80% of the blood volume is positioned below the heart. Thus, in response to reduced central blood volume, cardiovascular reflexes including sympathetic activation and the veno-arterial reflex are important for maintaining the upright position. Yet, it is not possible to remain upright without the muscle pump preventing the accumulation of blood in dependent parts of the body, as is the case in soldiers standing still in line who faint with a concomitant decrease in heart rate and blood pressure. This reflex, defined as *vasovagal syncope*, is elicited when central blood volume is reduced by 30% as a result of gravitational pooling in the upright posture, and the associated reduction in blood pressure is attributed to a *Bezold–Jarisch-like reflex* that induces vasodilatation in skeletal muscles at the expense of flow to the brain.

Starling's law of the heart

The influence of central blood volume, or cardiac preload, on the function of the heart is described by Starling's law of the heart (Fig. 4.12). In this context, *normovolemia*, defined by the absence of further increase in stroke volume or cardiac output when central blood volume increases, is achieved in the supine posture. During head-down tilt, which increases diastolic filling of the heart, there is no further stroke volume increase indicating that the upper flat part of the Starling curve has been reached. Conversely, when upright, central blood volume is

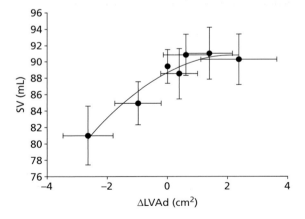

Fig. 4.12 Starling curve for the human heart as evaluated during head-up and head-down tilt. During supine rest the upper flat part of the curve is reached. SV, stroke volume, ΔLVAd, change in left ventricular diameter (Courtesy of Ø. Jans).

reduced and the heart operates on the ascending part of the Starling curve where cardiac output depends on preload.

During rowing, central blood volume and the ~10% increase in working muscles blood volume are supported by the muscle pump promoting venous return and the redistribution of blood volume by vasoconstriction in the splanchnic area. However, with increasing blood flow requirements in working muscles and the skin, as body temperature increases, splanchnic vasoconstriction does not recruit enough blood to maintain the central blood volume level established at seated or supine rest. Central blood volume contributes to the level of sympathoexcitation established as illustrated by the heart rate response. For example, at supine rest the heart rate may be 60 beats·min^{-1} and increases to 80 beats·min^{-1} when standing but decreases to 70 beats·min^{-1} during contraction of the legs. Muscle contractions increase sympathetic activity but the concomitant enhancement of central blood volume and central venous pressure by the muscle pump elicits a "paradoxical" reduction in sympathetic activity. Similarly, during running, a reduced central blood volume attenuates central venous pressure and distension of the atria, as reflected by the plasma level of atrial natriuretic peptide (ANP).

Consequently, heart rate is higher during running than during rowing at a given exercise $\dot{V}O_2$. Furthermore, the lowest heart rate response to exercise is observed in the supine posture. This gravitational influence on heart rate is sustained during maximal exercise, as indicated by the lower value during rowing than during running despite the larger $\dot{V}O_{2max}$ established by the larger active muscle mass during rowing. With the enhanced central blood volume following rowing training, heart rate at a given work load, including maximal effort, decreases.

Cardiac output

The cardiac output depends on the volume of blood that the heart receives, or its preload. As the total capacitance of the vasculature is larger than the total blood volume, the distribution of blood volume is critical for maintenance of blood pressure and regional flow. Blood volume encompasses both volumes of red cells and plasma which changes rapidly in response to rowing. For example, plasma volume is elevated by 20% following short-term training and it decreases during bed rest or during space flight. The enlargement of plasma volume following training, and the reduction in plasma volume when central blood volume remains elevated, demonstrate that central blood volume rather than total blood volume is the regulated variable.

During rowing, body weight is lost by sweating, but even after weight is restored by drinking, central blood volume remains reduced for many hours following rowing and plasma volume is expanded by further drinking as thirst is maintained. Central blood volume is reduced following rowing due to muscle edema provoked by the combined effects of elevated perfusion pressure and muscle vasodilatation associated with rowing. Also, cutaneous vasodilatation induced by the elevated body temperature contributes to the attenuation of central blood volume during and after rowing. Even though body temperature normalizes and muscle edema is cleared rapidly post-rowing, muscle blood volume is maintained elevated for almost a day and that volume is recruited from the central circulation, as detected by DLCO (Fig. 4.8) and thoracic electrical impedance.

The reduced central blood volume following rowing is reflected in the levels of hormones that regulate fluid balance, including plasma vasopressin (alternatively named antidiuretic hormone; ADH) and plasma ANP. Plasma vasopressin remains elevated while plasma ANP is low following rowing and both these hormonal changes reduce urine production resulting in positive fluid balance. It is less clear why the red cell volume increases in response to training. Bone marrow is stimulated by erythropoietin (EPO) released mainly from the kidneys to produce hemoglobin. Exposure to high altitude hypoxia increases hemoglobin production, but the acute increase in hematocrit reflects the loss of plasma volume. Rowing, in addition to the exercise-induced hypoxemia stimulus for EPO production, may stimulate hemoglobin production via the sympathetically induced reduction in kidney blood flow, a mechanism similar to the low EPO production and associated anemia observed in kidney diseases.

Table 4.2 Hemoglobin, hematocrit, red blood cells, plasma volume and blood volume in male sedentary population and in elite male rowers.

	Sedentary	Elite rower
Hemoglobin (g·L^{-1})	150	165
Hematocrit (%)	43	48
Red blood cells (L)	2.4	3.1
Plasma volume (L)	3.2	4.8
Blood volume (L)	5.0	7.2

The increase in total hemoglobin is an important adaptation to training because $\dot{V}O_{2max}$ is related to red cell volume rather than to the hemoglobin concentration. In a seeming paradox, despite the increased red cell volume, elite rowers often present low hemoglobin concentrations (or hematocrit), as a result of the training-induced enlarged plasma volume. For elite rowers, plasma and red cell volume may be 4.8 and 3.1 L, respectively, compared with reference values of 3.2 and 2.4 L, respectively, for controls. Yet, on average, the hemoglobin concentration of rowers is larger than for the normal healthy population (see Fig. 11.3) (Table 4.2).

The heart

As known from cardiac diseases, the heart adapts to the load it is exposed to and that adaptation also applies to training. With endurance training the internal diameters of the heart enlarge, with the highest values observed in professional bicyclists with 55 versus 50 mL for untrained subjects. The heart of weightlifters is different because they develop high blood pressure during each maximal effort by a concomitantly performed Valsalva-like maneuver which stabilizes the spine. To overcome the high blood pressure, the wall thickness of the heart's septum separating the left and right ventricle increases to 10 mm, while the internal diameters of the heart remain unchanged.

In rowing and kayaking, as in many other activities, there is a combined demand for a large $\dot{V}O_{2max}$, cardiac output and stroke volume in addition to overcoming the high blood pressure at the beginning of each rowing stroke. It follows that both the

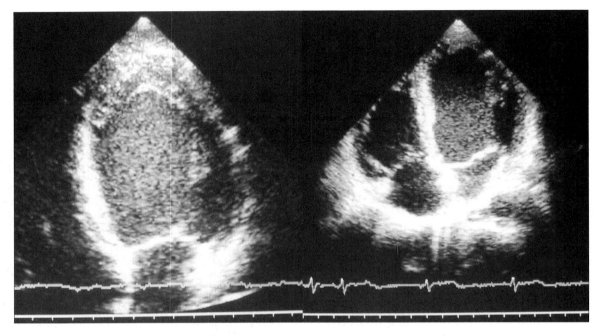

Fig. 4.13 Echocardiographic presentation of the heart in diastole of a World champion rower (left) and a control subject (right) of similar size. For the rower, the internal diameter of the left ventricle is 6.4 cm compared to 4.9 cm for the control subject. Similarly, the septum has a width of 1.3 and 0.8 cm, respectively, and the posterior wall of the heart a width of 1.2 and 0.9 cm, respectively. Courtesy of Emma Hart, Brunel University.

internal dimensions and wall thickness of the heart increase and elite rowers possess the largest sports heart with values for left ventricular mass of 330 g compared with 142 g for divers (Fig. 4.13).

About 7% of elite rowers have both a left ventricular wall thickness over the normal limit of 13 mm and an enlarged left ventricular cavity. In elite rowers, the heart is so enlarged that myocardial perfusion becomes inhomogeneous, which together with high vagal tone and low intrinsic heart rate (after combined vagal and sympathetic blockade), creates a complicated electrocardiographic presentation. As in skeletal muscles, training increases capillarization of the heart and following detraining, the size of the heart returns to its control values.

While it is difficult to maintain an adequate preload to the heart during seated and especially upright exercise, there is little problem for the heart to pump the blood it is provided with. In contrast to the pain experienced in skeletal muscles during sustained rowing, healthy people do not complain of chest pain during rowing, indicating that myocardial oxygen demand does not limit cardiac output. Furthermore, it is energy-efficient for the heart to provide a large cardiac output.

Energy requirements of the heart depend on its rate and (systolic) pressure expressed as the rate–pressure product. Following rowing training, the enlarged blood volume ensures filling of the heart and reduces sympathetic activity which attenuates heart rate by the same mechanism observed during supine and seated exercise. Furthermore, the enhanced central blood volume attenuates the pressure that arterial baroreceptors control during rowing, as exemplified by the blood pressure reduction when leg exercise is added to arm cranking. Cardiac output is elevated following rowing training with no additional strain on the heart (i.e., same rate–pressure product during maximal rowing),

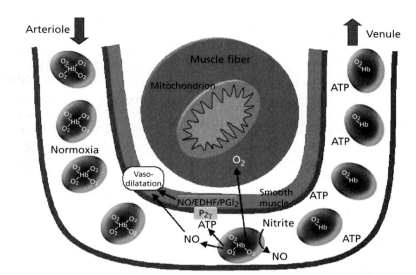

Fig. 4.14 Red cells passing through a capillary with substances released to dilatate the vessels as oxygen is liberated. ATP, adenosine triphosphate; EDHF, endothelia-derived-hyperpolarization-factor; Hb, hemoglobin; NO, nitric oxide; PGI$_2$, prostaglandin-2. Courtesy of Jose Gonzalez-Alonso, Brunel University.

indicating that the enhanced blood flow to active muscles is provided by means of enhanced vascular dilatation (Fig. 4.14). Yet, the muscle pump cannot provide enough blood to the heart and sometimes at exhaustion a restrain on cardiac preload is illustrated by decreasing central venous pressure.

Stroke volume

The stroke volume of elite rowers is impressive (195 versus 110 mL for control subjects), but it is not limited by the capacity of the heart to encompass a large volume of blood. The problem upright humans face in increasing cardiac output during exercise is different from that experienced by quadrupedal animals. In puppies, exercise capacity increases following pericardiectomy which allows the heart to expand. In upright humans, there is not a similar restrain on stoke volume as illustrated by the filling of the heart during supine exercise and by the ability of the heart to increase stroke volume in response to a volume overload. With administration of the plasma expander Macrodex® heart rate during maximal exercise decreases (183 versus 188 beats·min^{-1}) while stroke volume is enhanced by 10% (155–144 mL).

Following volume expansion, the enhanced stroke volume confirms that the heart operates at the ascending part of the Starling curve when humans are upright. The size of the heart remains unchanged and it may decrease somewhat when heart rate exceeds 150 beats·min^{-1}, indicating that the heart propels the blood it is provided with. During rowing, stroke volume increases by enhanced contractility and the systolic duration shortens to about half while the diastolic duration is further limited to one-third of the resting value. Exercise tachycardia develops although plasma potassium increases (e.g., to 6–7 mmol·L^{-1}), signifying that sympathetic activation is needed not only to maintain function of the heart but also to clear plasma potassium during and after rowing.

The short diastolic interval during rowing may present a problem for the filling of the heart as illustrated in patients with atrial fibrillation where cardiac output is compromised when heart rate exceeds 120 beats·min^{-1}. However, during rowing, venous return is enhanced and increased contractility of the heart is important. Sympathetic activation is supported by a small increase in free plasma calcium released from albumin as pH decreases. Relaxation of the left ventricle may draw blood into the heart and this action is enhanced when the end-systolic volume is attenuated during vigorous rowing. Yet, the attenuated heart rate response to rowing following training is an advantageous adaptation for the filling of the heart.

Extreme exercise

The ability of the heart to cope is less impressive during extreme exercise. Reports on horses running to death are not uncommon. It is also well-known that Pheidippides died after running the original Marathon course to report to Athens the Greek victory over the Persians (battle of Marathon, 490 BC) (it may be noted that previously he had been fighting in the battle after running 2×250 km (!) in a round trip from Athens to Sparta to request support). While running to exhaustion, the heart of rats is dilated and the blood volume encompassed within the cavities is elevated by 50% and normalizes only over days. That degree of exhaustion is further characterized by a state simulating thyroid insufficiency as illustrated by rats forced to swim to exhaustion which reduce their spontaneous activity, eat more and increase body weight.

The extent that the post-exercise stress syndrome in rats relates to overtraining in humans is only a speculation, but long distance events such as long distance rowing or rowing marathons provoke cardiac fatigue. Cardiac fatigue is presented primarily as reduced diastolic function of the heart. Both chronotropic and inotropic functions are affected by competitions lasting many hours as illustrated by attenuated responses to sympathomimetic drugs (e.g., by beta-receptor down-regulation or desensitization).

Cardiac output

In 1920, cardiac output was measured during rowing in fixed-seat rowing boats by Liljestrand and Lindhard, showing values of 13–17 L·min^{-1} and reached up to ~30 L·min^{-1} in lightweight rowers during ergometer rowing. Cardiac output provides blood flow to tissues including working skeletal muscles and there is, on average, a 7.3 : 1 coupling between cardiac output and $\dot{V}_{O_2}$ in untrained humans or 6.5 : 1 in trained rowers. The largest reported $\dot{V}_{O_2max}$ of 7.4 L·min^{-1} would thereby be expected to require a cardiac output of 49 L·min^{-1} and values of 40 L·min^{-1} are reported regularly. There are, however, large inter-individual variations in cardiac output both at rest and during rowing. At rest, some variation relates to body size and cardiac output is expressed as cardiac index

(3.5 L·min^{-1}·m^{-2}) in cardiology with body surface area based on height and weight (~1.7 m^2). During exercise, cardiac output values usually range 29–40 L·min^{-1}, with the highest values achieved by those athletes who present also large body size: height exceeding 199 cm, body mass around 90 kg, body fat percent below 9%, $\dot{V}_{O_2max}$ higher than 6.7 L·min^{-1} and average $\dot{V}_{O_2}$ consumption during a 2000 m simulated rowing race at least 98% of $\dot{V}_{O_2max}$ (Table 4.1). Additionally, cardiac output varies according to the variation in genes, as demonstrated by the arg16gly polymorphism of the β_2-adrenergic receptor, and with hematocrit.

During rowing, pulmonary $\dot{V}_{O_2}$ increases in relation to metabolism in exercising muscles with oxygen uptake of non-exercising tissues being 0.4 L·min^{-1}. Such observations underscore a tight coupling between cardiac output, regional blood flow and metabolism with some attenuation of blood flow at the highest workloads. Yet, it is not blood flow per se that is regulated but rather oxygen-carrying capacity defined as venous oxygen saturation because red cells liberate vasodilatating substances when they release oxygen (Fig. 4.14).

The postulate of an oxygen-dependent regulation of cardiac output and regional blood flow assumes that the heart provides the needed cardiac output but this is not always the case. When the circulating blood volume is reduced, as exemplified by sweating during prolonged rowing or dehydration, cardiac output is smaller than expected according to hematocrit.

Blood pressure

Arterial pressure has two roles in the regulation of blood flow to tissues. Arterial pressure is the key regulated circulatory variable controlled beat by beat from the arterial baroreceptors which modulate peripheral resistance and blood pressure serves for perfusion pressure to the tissues and notably to the brain. Thus, cerebral blood flow is dependent on mean arterial pressure. At rest, variation in blood pressure is related to the cardiac cycle, resulting in a pulse pressure of approximately 45 mmHg. During rowing, however, blood pressure also varies with the rowing cycle, giving rise to a "pulse pressure" of

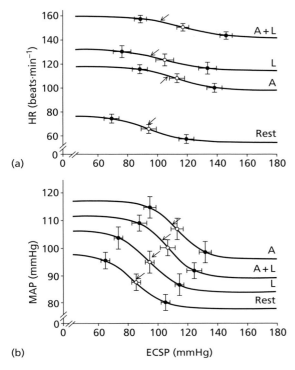

(a)

(b)

ECSP (mmHg)

Fig. 4.15 The carotid baroreflex during arm (A), leg (L) and combined arm and leg exercise (A + L). At rest the actual pressure (arrow) corresponds to the maximum gain of the reflex (o), while during exercise it may be positioned at a slightly lower estimated carotid sinus pressure (ECSP) suggesting that the baroreflex detects hypotension although blood pressure is elevated. HR, heart rate; MAP, mean arterial pressure.

more than 100 mmHg because of the Valsalva-like maneuver performed at the catch of each stroke. This means that the systolic pressure may approach 200 mmHg during maximal rowing. Regulation of arterial pressure by the arterial baroreceptors during rowing implies that their operating range is right-shifted and elevated by neural influence from central command and *the muscle pressor reflex* (Fig. 4.15).

Two strategies may be applied to establish the elevated pressure that the baroreceptors are reset to control. Ideally, the set pressure can be established by an increase in cardiac output to compensate for the marked decrease in total peripheral resistance induced by rowing. However, if that is not possible because of strain on cardiac output either by a restricted preload or by an inability of the heart to

produce the required cardiac output, mean arterial pressure is maintained by vasoconstriction not only to internal organs but also to working muscles and to the brain.

Regional blood flow

Skeletal muscle blood flow is modulated by deoxy-genation of hemoglobin adjusting flow to metabolism and that takes place despite the enhanced sympathetic activity during rowing (Fig. 4.14). Such sympatholysis depends also on other factors such as the elevated muscle temperature, potassium, nitric oxide and the arterial pyruvate : lactate ratio. However, muscle blood flow is not allowed to increase at the expense of blood pressure.

Priority for blood pressure regulation over regulation of flow is demonstrated when comparison is made between flow to a muscle working in isolation and together with other muscles. As an example, flow to working legs (~10 L·min⁻¹) is reduced when the arms are working intensely at the same time. Equally, arm blood flow (4.6 L·min⁻¹ in untrained vs. 6.4 L·min⁻¹ in rowers) and oxygenation are larger during arm cranking than when arm cranking is performed together with high intensity cycling exercise (Fig. 4.16).

Skeletal muscles seldom receive the blood flow that their vasculature can handle. During rowing especially, flow to the working muscles is reduced by ~20–40% compared to the flow they receive during exercise involving small muscle mass, and this reduction is manifested primarily via sympathetically mediated enhanced vascular resistance. However, when leg exercise is added to arm cranking, blood pressure decreases and perfusion pressure to the arm accounts for approximately 50% of the reduction in arm blood flow.

Muscles

The final step in the oxygen transport chain to muscle is by diffusion. Capillaries are recruited when muscles are activated, suggesting that the capillary network is designed to provide the muscle

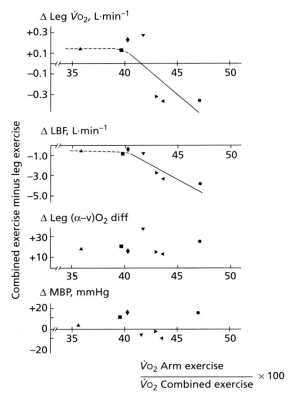

Fig. 4.16 Effect of adding arm exercise to leg exercise on leg oxygen uptake ($\dot{V}O_2$), leg blood flow (LBF), the leg arterial to venous oxygen difference [(a–v)O_2 diff], and mean arterial pressure (MAP).

with oxygen during rowing rather than at rest. In fact, arteries are not gas impermeable and a considerable amount of gas exchange (oxygen uptake and elimination of CO_2) takes place in vessels larger than the capillaries. Yet, during rowing, muscle cells are provided with oxygen through diffusion from the capillaries. There is a coupling between $\dot{V}O_{2max}$ and capillary density and more capillaries surround ST and FT muscle fibers. Typical values for the vastus lateralis muscle are 1.8 capillaries per fiber for untrained and 2.6 capillaries per fiber for trained rowers while the highest capillarization is observed in the internal intercostal muscles with 6 capillaries per fiber.

As with the lungs, the oxygen diffusion capacity of the muscles can be calculated. As with the lungs, the available oxygen diffusion capacity of the muscles is not always used. During moderate rowing, capillary recruitment enhances the gas diffusion capacity, but during maximal rowing blood flow is limited and thus gas diffusion is restrained. During arm only exercise, gas diffusion values of the arm may be 20 and $50\,mL\cdot min^{-1}\cdot mmHg^{-1}$ in untrained and trained rowers, respectively, while it decreases to $32\,mL\cdot min^{-1}\cdot mmHg^{-1}$ when legwork is added to arm only exercise.

Brain

Ultimately, it is the brain that limits performance. Central fatigue was described by the Italian physiologist A. Mosso (1904). Using a finger ergograph he demonstrated that fatigue becomes pronounced after a demanding mental task such as a lecture. Since the work of Mosso, central fatigue has been described in a wide range of situations and, conversely, the enhanced performance associated with so-called diverting activities may be seen as alleviating that type of fatigue. The influence of diverting activities on muscle fatigue (Setchenov's phenomenon) refers to the observation that performance is enhanced when exercise with one muscle group (e.g., with one hand) is supplemented by activity with another muscle group. Similarly, if exercise is continued until exhaustion with the eyes closed, opening of the eyes enhances strength and work can be continued for some time.

Another delineation of a limitation to recruitment of muscles is the varying strength established when contractions are performed with either one or both legs (Fig. 4.17). The force developed during simultaneous contraction of the legs is less than the sum of strength developed during contractions of one leg at a time and this "leg strength paradox" is modulated by training. Walking and running are characterized by alternative use of the legs (i.e., one leg is extending while the other leg is flexing), whereas in rowing both legs are used concomitantly to apply force on the foot-stretchers. Likely for that reason, rowers are able to develop strength while using both legs that is equal to, or exceeds, the sum of the strength that they are able to develop with one leg.

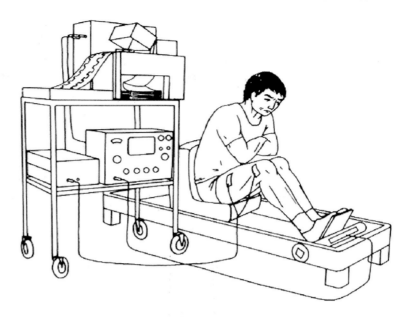

Fig. 4.17 Experimental set-up and evaluation of leg strength.

The ability to resist fatigue is enhanced by training and this effect is, moreover, so specific that to a large extent it must be ascribed to the enhanced ability to recruit motoneurons. Training of repeated one-legged contractions postpones, as expected, onset of fatigue during one-legged contractions while performance with both legs remains unchanged (Fig. 4.18). Conversely, training the extension of both legs benefits contractions involving both legs, whereas the performance of one leg is, surprisingly, unchanged and, under both circumstances, the electromyographic activity over the muscles decreases in parallel with force. Also, after maximal dynamic exercise, central fatigue is important as demonstrated by electrical stimulation of the motoneuron that yields a greater power than that evoked by voluntary contractions. Finally, the consistent finding that a ~25% increase in strength takes place without hypertrophy of the muscle fibers confirms that full recruitment of muscle fibers requires a central adaptation or a learning process.

With varying ability of the central nervous system to recruit the motoneurons, the pattern of muscle contractions developed during central fatigue is of interest. During partial neuromuscular blockade, two types of contractions can be delineated. With the use of an acetylcholine agonist drug (decamethonium or suxamethonium), muscle contractions become slow but enduring. Conversely, a nondepolarizing neuromuscular blocking agent (e.g., tubocurarine) provokes contractions that maintain a high rate of rise of tension, but the developed force fades off rapidly. Because the two types of neuromuscular blocking agents affect selectively fast and slow twitch fibers, respectively, the contraction pattern manifested during partial neuromuscular blockade provides some insight into the characteristics of the two main fiber types in humans. From that perspective, it seems that central fatigue affects the recruitment of slow rather than fast twitch muscle fibers as the contraction maintains its rate of rise of tension and, at the same time, loses its endurance (Fig. 4.19).

The central nervous system mechanisms responsible for central fatigue remain elusive. One consideration relevant to central fatigue is that stimulation of cortical areas provokes facilitation of reflexes over fast muscles and, conversely, inhibits reflexes involving slow muscles. In the following, the cerebral metabolic response to exercise will be addressed from the perspective that central fatigue may be provoked by a limited provision of oxygen and substrate to relevant areas of the brain.

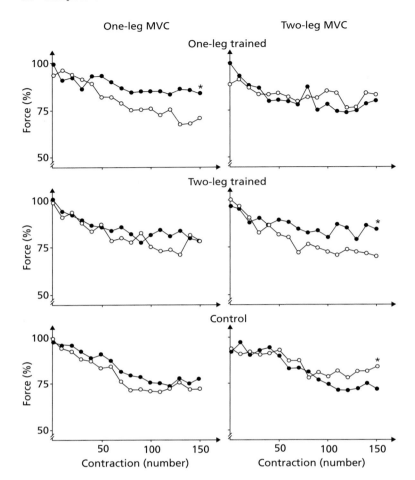

Fig. 4.18 Fatigue during repeated one- and two-legged contractions following one- or two-legged training. MVC, maximum voluntary contraction.

Cerebral blood flow during exercise

While demonstration of central fatigue during different human activities may seem trivial, it has been a challenge to identify changes within the brain that correlate to hampered recruitment of the muscles. With physical activity regional cerebral blood flow (CBF) increases in activated areas of the brain but, for the brain as a whole, there is not much, if any increase in CBF. A stable global CBF during exercise may imply that increased activity in one cerebral region is compensated by down-regulation in other regions, and may explain why it is difficult to do more than one concentrated effort at a time. Furthermore, with the marked hyperventilation associated with maximal whole body exercise such as rowing, the arterial carbon dioxide

tension decreases and that reduces CBF. Together with the hypoxemia developed during rowing (arterial oxygen saturation decreasing from 97% to 90%), the reduction in CBF means that cerebral oxygenation decreases by ~10%. Such a reduction in cerebral oxygenation is significant because it is of the same magnitude as seen during fainting and therefore a likely contributing factor to central fatigue.

Cerebral energy metabolism

Changes in brain metabolism are expressed by the ratio of oxygen to carbohydrate uptake of the brain, known as the cerebral metabolic ratio (MR), which at rest is close to 6. Cerebral metabolism depends primarily on oxidation of carbohydrate as the brain

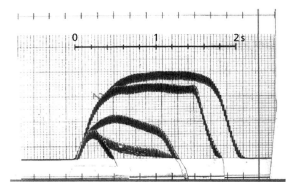

Fig. 4.19 Registration of force during repeated maximal voluntary handgrip contractions. As force decreases, also the ability to maintain the contraction becomes affected, while there is little reduction in the rate of rise of tension. Thus, at exhaustion, the contraction has a duration of ~0.3 s, while the normal maximal contraction lasts for some 2–3 s. During partial neuromuscular blockade by tubocuarine, rate of tension is similarly maintained, while the developed force fades off after 0.15 s to continue at a much lower level after ~0.3 s. Conversely, after the use of decamethonium or suxamethonium, the rate of rise of tension is affected severely, but the developed force can be maintained for as long as desired.

uptake of amino acids and free fatty acids is of little quantitative importance. During brain activation, however, MR decreases and, in that respect, physical exercise represents an extreme. The largest reduction in MR is established during exhaustive whole body exercise while MR increases to ~6.5 during anesthesia (Fig. 4.20). With intense ergometer rowing-induced activation of the brain, MR decreases to values lower than 2 suggesting less than 30% of the carbohydrate taken up by the brain is oxidized, or that up to ~10 mmol glucose-equivalents need to be accounted for.

For evaluation of MR during exercise, lactate is important. During resting wakefulness, the brain releases small amounts of lactate. In contrast, when exercise provokes a substantial increase in blood lactate, there is an uptake by the brain that is proportional to the arterial concentration. Seemingly, the lactate taken up by the brain is metabolized both by neurons and astrocytes as it is not accumulating within the cerebrospinal fluid or within the brain tissue. Breakdown of MR during exercise, however, does not depend on the lactate taken up by the brain. During prolonged exercise, there

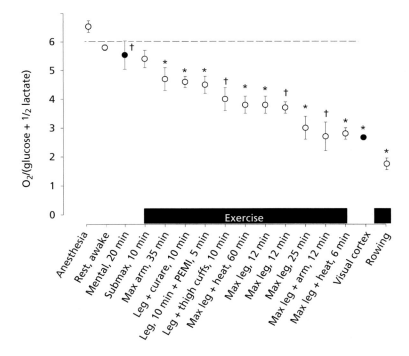

Fig. 4.20 The cerebral metabolic ratio (brain uptake of oxygen relative to that of carbohydrate; glucose + 1/2 lactate) during general anesthesia, at rest and during various types of brain activation including several types of exercise with ergometer rowing demonstrating the largest deviation from the resting value of 6.

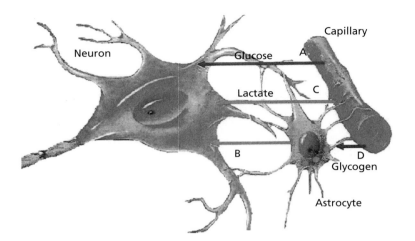

Fig. 4.21 Lactate from the blood and the astrocytes is taken up by activated neurons.

is only a modest or no increase in blood lactate and, accordingly, little lactate uptake by the brain. Yet MR decreases at exhaustion during prolonged exercise as during intense exercise of shorter duration.

Brain glycogen metabolism

During muscle contractions, part of the energy is derived from glycogen breakdown and during sustained muscle work fatigue presents when glycogen deposits are depleted. Similarly, the brain glycogen level decreases during neuronal activity. The human brain glycogen concentration is ~6 mmol·L^{-1} (glucosyl units) in gray and white matter and as high as 13 mmol·L^{-1} in the hippocampus. Therefore, the total glycogen content in the brain is estimated to be ~10 mmol·L^{-1}. In the brain, glycogen is confined primarily to the astrocytes; thus, the intracellular concentration of glycogen in the astrocytes may approach that of skeletal muscle, underpinning its potential importance as a fast accessible energy reservoir (Fig. 4.21).

In analogy with skeletal muscle, central fatigue could be provoked when the brain glycogen level reaches a critically low level, and the "extra" and unaccounted for carbohydrate uptake by the brain could have a role during such energetic imbalance. By provoking such a crisis during exercise in hypoxia, isometric contractions become more affected than fast contractions, suggesting that recruitment of slow twitch fibers is more vulnerable to central fatigue than that of fast twitch muscle fibers. If so, central fatigue represents an exception to the normal "orderly recruitment" of muscle fibers where slow twitch fibers are recruited before fast twitch muscle fibers. Inability to maintain slow twitch muscle fiber recruitment explains why fatigue manifests as difficulty in preserving a smooth movement.

Also brain temperature is important and work is stopped when its temperature reaches 40–41°C. Conversely, proper hydration allows for evaporation of water and control of temperature while training may be interpreted as preparation of the cardiorespiratory system to provide oxygen and substrates to working muscles so that work can be carried out without the brain being aware of the effort. Taken together, the cardiorespiratory system has the capacity to increase $\dot{V}O_{2max}$ by modulating each of the different steps in the transport system with the exception of the pulmonary system as the only organ for which adaptation to endurance training has not been demonstrated.

References and recommended reading

Dalsgaard, M.K. (2006) Fuelling cerebral activity in exercising man. *Journal of Cerebral Blood Flow and Metabolism* **26**, 731–750.

Ide, K. & Secher, N.H. (2000) Cerebral blood flow and metabolism during exercise. *Progress in Neurobiology* **61**, 397–414.

Jensen, K., Johansen, L. & Secher, N.H. (2001) Influence on body mass on maximal oxygen uptake, effect of sample size. *European Journal of Applied Physiology* **84**, 201–205.

Mosso, A. (1904) *Fatigue*. Swan Sonnenschein, London.

Nybo, L. & Secher, N.H. (2004) Cerebral perturbations provoked by prolonged exercise. *Progress in Neurobiology* **72**, 223–261.

Secher, N.H. (1983) The physiology of rowing. *Journal of Sports Sciences* **1**, 23–53.

Secher, N.H. & Volianitis, S. (2006) Are the arms and legs in competition for cardiac output? *Medicine and Science in Sports and Exercise* **38**, 1797–1803.

Volianitis, S., McConnell, A.K., Koutedakis, Y., McNaughton, L., Backx, K. & Jones, D.A. (2001) Inspiratory muscle training improves rowing performance. *Medicine and Science in Sports and Exercise* **33**, 803–809.

Wagner, P.D., Hoppler, H. & Saltin, B. (1977) Determinants of maximal oxygen uptake. In: R.G. Crystal & J.B. West (eds) *The Lung*. Lippincott-Raven, Philadelphia. pp. 2033–2041.

Chapter 5
Overtraining

S. Volianitis and H.B. Nielsen

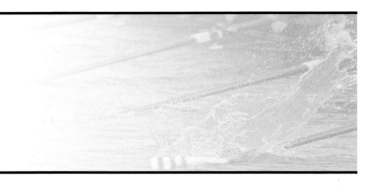

Introduction

Training adaptation depends on the athlete's physiologic and psychologic responses to four important training factors: type, frequency, duration and intensity of exercise, which, unless they are managed carefully, can lead to overtraining (Chapter 7). Following each training session a catabolic phase with decreased tolerance of effort develops, characterized by reversible biochemical, hormonal and immunologic changes. An anabolic phase with a higher adaptive capacity and enhanced performance capacity follows. Failing to adapt to training has some major physiologic and psychologic consequences, all of which lead to increasingly poorer training and competitive performances. It is difficult to assess the relative impact of training on the athlete and there seem to be no specific preliminary symptoms to warn the athlete of failing adaptation. An optimal training program therefore needs an adequate assessment of the current individual tolerance to stress which can be affected not only by training and competitions, but also by disease and injury as well as professional and social stressors.

Definitions and symptoms

An imbalance between the overall strain and the current tolerance to stress leads to failure of training adaptation and overtraining. Short-term overtraining is called overreaching, and can be reversed by a more prolonged period of regeneration. It is difficult to distinguish between failing to adapt to training (overtraining) and chronic fatigue resulting from training (overreaching). The day-to-day variations in the sensation of fatigue should not be confused with failing adaptation. Chronic fatigue can result from consecutive days or bouts of hard training or intense competition but can be relieved with a few days of easy training, no competition and a carbohydrate-rich diet.

Further exposure to stressors will induce an overtraining syndrome or "staleness" for a prolonged period (i.e., more than 2 weeks). Symptoms of failing adaptation vary among individuals but the most common general feeling is heaviness in the muscles. This is usually accompanied by a gradual deterioration in training and competitive performances. At present, there are no early clear warning signs, or body alarm systems, that indicate a failure to adapt to training and by the time failing adaptation has been recognized, it is usually too late to effectively reverse the condition and the athlete's only option is weeks or months of reduced training or complete rest which could mean the end of high level competition for that year. Most symptoms are subjective and identifiable only after athletes have overextended themselves. Athletes who suddenly begin to produce extraordinary training performances may get excited about these performances and overextend themselves by training at a greater than normal intensity and duration, and thus overtrain.

With the onset of failing adaptation, the athlete usually experiences a vicious cycle in trying to overcome the poor training and competitive performances by training harder or changing technique. These responses often lead to even greater physical and physiologic deterioration and psychologic frustration. The athlete, at this point, is uncertain about his or her skill and, in many cases, loses confidence. In addition, increasing training effort or changing technique can lead to serious injury that may prevent the athlete from competing to their potential.

The more advanced so-called parasympathicotonic form of the overtraining syndrome is typically associated with less obvious symptoms, while the predominantly sympathicotonic form of the overtraining syndrome is easier to recognize because of more pronounced vegetative complaints. A mixture of these two forms often exists, because the sympathicotonic type represents an early transient stage shifting to the parasympathicotonic after varied periods of time. Generally, overtraining is characterized by a decreased sports-specific performance capacity and pronounced vegetative complaints, such as altered psychic excitability, sleep disorders, emotional instability and organ-related complaints without organic disease.

A critical aspect of failing adaptation is that it is often the most highly skilled and motivated athlete who is susceptible to failing adaptation (Chapter 6). Those prone to overtraining are excessively aggressive athletes who are always trying to perform at their best, are more critical of themselves than others, have set extremely high standards, want to win at all costs, and cannot seem to get enough work. Failing adaptation is difficult to define and even more difficult to measure and prevent.

Typical symptoms of overtraining syndrome

• Impaired mood profile: increased fatigue, increased depression
• Increased subjective rating of effort
• Decreased maximal anaerobic lactic capacity
• Often unaltered submaximal lactate–performance relationship
• Higher heart rate at rest and during submaximal exercise an early sign of infectious disease

Specific symptoms

Physical and physiologic

1 Excessive and unusual weight loss
2 Change in body composition; decrease in body fat
3 Decreased appetite
4 Local muscular tiredness and heaviness
5 Sleep disturbances
6 Elevated heart rate, blood pressure and core temperature
7 Decrease in immune protection
8 Decrease in male and female sex hormones
9 Overworking

Psychologic

1 Frustration
2 Loss of confidence
3 Wide mood swings
4 Uncommunicative and quiet
5 Self-pity
6 Tardiness and missing workouts
7 Depression
8 Anxiety
9 Trying too hard
10 Inability to relax

Factors inducing overtraining

During rowing at intensities below the lactate threshold, there is no rise in blood lactate levels and only a little sympathetic activity is to be expected. In contrast, prolonged training performed at intensities exceeding the lactate threshold is characterized by a disproportionate increase of stress hormones (free epinephrine and norepinephrine) concentration, thus limiting the frequency of such training sessions. Repetitive training with high lactate concentrations, and thus high adrenergic stimulation, probably represents the most dangerous form of exercise which could eventually induce an overtraining syndrome. In a 2-year study, involving 17 endurance trained athletes, overtraining was induced mainly by an increase in training intensity.

Training plans should also consider the technical skills of the rowers. For example, two rowers with uneven skills can have different lactate–performance curves determined in the boat despite very similar curves determined on the ergometer. Thus, training prescription oriented only on heart rate measurements during ergometric tests would lead to different training effects and eventually to overtraining of one rower, while the other rower would exercise in an adequate or even insufficient range of intensity.

When considering the exercise tolerance of athletes, not only the training but also the specific stress during competition is to be considered, which cannot be objectively determined by metabolic measurements such as blood lactate concentrations. Psychologic stress during competitive events is characterized by a higher catecholamines:lactate ratio in comparison to training exercise sessions. In many cases, the overtraining syndrome has not been induced by competition or training, but by the addition of other stress factors, such as a period of examinations in students, or insufficient recovery after infectious diseases, when the coach or athlete fears loosing time from training.

Although the causes for deterioration in performance are not clear, it appears that intensity of training imposes greater stress than either duration or frequency of training. There is also evidence suggesting that factors unrelated to training such as job or school related, social, economic or personal problems may be partially responsible for failing adaptation. Several physiologic and physical causes of overtraining have been suggested:

1 Rapid increase in training intensity and/or volume; it is suggested that less than 1% increase per week for intensity and 3–5% per week for volume be used
2 Chronic damage to muscle cells; death of cells
3 Overload of immune system
4 Abnormal endocrine responses
5 Disruption of connective tissue; tendon and ligament destruction
6 Nutrient deficiency: vitamins, minerals, etc.
7 Depletion of energy sources: glycogen, fats
8 Red blood cell damage and destruction
9 Chronic dehydration; decrease in blood volume

10 Anorexia nervosa
11 Abnormal cardiac rhythms
12 Decreased liver function
13 Chronic elevation of core temperature

Possible psychologic causes, like the physiologic and physical causes, are linked closely to the many symptoms listed. The continued erosion of confidence, overworking in response to ever-decreasing training and competitive performances, and constant frustration are a few of the important psychologic causes of failing adaptation.

The immune response and blood clotting

The immune system provides defense against viral, bacteria and cancer cells and includes both physical barriers (the skin, the airway mucosa, etc.) and immunocompetent cells in the tissues including blood. The immunocompetent cells in blood are characterized according to cell surface markers (CD) that describe the cell function. The hematopoietic stem cells, from which all blood cells are derived, have the cell surface marker CD34. The white blood cells or the leukocytes are separated into lymphocytes and granulocytes. The granulocytes are in turn divided into neutrophil, eosinophil and basophil cells according to their staining characteristics. Each white blood cell line has its defined role in the defense against what the immune system recognizes as foreign.

Lymphocytes are the main cell type in lymph nodes and in response to a throat infection, for example, lymphocytes accumulate in the lymph nodes to fight an infection brought forward from an infected area by the lymph. Thus, a throat infection manifests with swollen and tender lymph nodes along the neck musculature. Similarly, an infected blister on the hand may be complicated by fever and red lymph vessels along the length of the arm besides swollen lymph glands under the arm (blood poisoning) and that situation should be treated immediately by revision of the infected site by antibiotics.

The lymphocytes are divided into T cells, which respond primarily to viral infections, and B cells, of which the plasma cells produce immuno-globulins against bacteria. Both cell types are part of the memory of the immune system which following exposure to an infectious agent up-regulates and attenuates the effect of subsequent exposure. This characteristic of the immune system forms the basis for vaccination against infectious diseases.

Lymphocytes are CD3 positive and the T cells are either CD4 positive (T helper cells) or CD8 positive (T suppressor cells), but a minor portion of the cells may be positive for both CD4 and CD8. The B cells bear the CD19 marker. Some of the lymphocytes do not express CD3 and are named natural killer (NK) cells with CD16 and CD56 cell markers. In blood these cells constitute about 5–10% of lymphocytes and represent the first line of defense against viral and some cancer cells.

Importantly, the neurotrophil granulocyte gener-ates the inflammation response as when a blister becomes infected. A blister is most often infected with the staphylococcus bacteria normally found on the skin, and neurotrophil granulocytes migrate to the area to attack the bacteria and the skin becomes red, swollen and tender. In addition, the activity of the neurotrophil granulocytes generates the cellular debris that can be extracted from the infected area. The eosinophil cells respond to allergy and, as for the mast cells, histamine is released when these cells are activated. Histamine provokes symp-toms from the airways and in the skin; a rash devel-ops as following a mosquito sting, the so-called type IV response of the immune system.

With respect to rowing, interest in the immune system has centered on the observation that there appears to be an increased incidence of upper respi-ratory tract infections following strenuous exercise. An early finding was that exercise increases the number of leukocytes in blood and an increased eosinophil cell count was described even in the preparation for the Harvard–Yale Boat Race. An important question has been whether the immune system is suppressed in the hours following intense exercise and in particular after rowing. Following strenuous exercise, the function of the cellular immune system may be suppressed and make the rower vulnerable to micro-organisms (*the open window theory*).

Lymphocyte count, subpopulations and natural killer cells

Lymphocytes are found in blood and in lymphoid tissue including the lymph nodes and the spleen, and lymphocytes circulate between blood and the pulp of the spleen. During exercise the size of the spleen, influenced from the sympathetic nervous system, is reduced markedly in animals and in humans, accounting for one-fourth of the hemo-concentration associated with exercise. During intense rowing, the increase in plasma catecho-lamines also contributes to the several-fold increased release of lymphocytes from the spleen into the blood steam. In the first 2–4 h after maximal rowing, however, the lymphocyte count decreases to, or below, the pre-exercise level, probably by reuptake in the spleen.

During rowing, the relative contribution of the $CD4^+$ and $CD8^+$ T cells does not follow the increase in the total lymphocyte count. Only the fraction of the $CD16^+/CD56^+$ NK cells that represents the first line of defense against infection becomes elevated. Considering the change from the resting level, the concentration of NK cells increases markedly and a pronounced response is established during a 6-min maximal ergometer row (Fig. 5.1).

Thus, the blood concentration of both lym-phocyte T and B cells increases significantly during maximal rowing. The increased concentration of T cells is established as both the concentration of memory and the virgin T cells become elevated. The increase in white blood cell concentrations during and after rowing reflects redistribution of cells rather than activation of the immune system.

Lymphocyte function

NK cell activity increases during rowing but follow-ing exercise the activity returns to the resting level or decreases. Such suppression of the NK cell activ-ity is most pronounced within 2–4 h after exercise. During maximal rowing, a discrepancy between the increase in the percentage of NK cells and that in the average NK cell activity is established suggesting that the activity of each NK cell is suppressed. Accordingly, it seems that either the functional capacity of each NK cell is reduced in response to

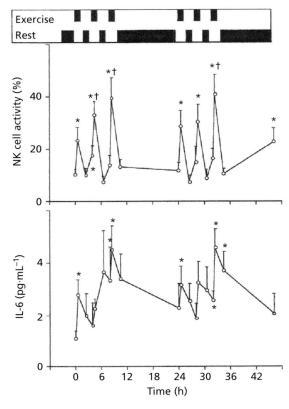

Fig. 5.1 Natural killer (NK) cell activity response to repeated bouts of maximal ergometer rowing over 2 days. Also shown the interleukin-6 (IL-6) response. IL-6 is a cytokine that is released from muscles and the brain in response to an energy "crises". * Different from rest; † Different from first row.

rowing, or cells with smaller than average activity are recruited from the spleen. Yet, if the activity of the NK cells is reduced after rowing, it would be considered to be of little practical consequence because of the small contribution of the NK cells to the total immune response. In support of that view, it is found that after exposure to a rhinovirus, the severity of a cold is not greater in people who have been exercising than in a control group of subjects.

Immunoglobulins

The functional capacity of lymphocyte B cells is evaluated by assessment of immunoglobulins (Ig)

in serum or *in vitro* following a proliferative response. There are five lines of immunoglobulins (IgA, IgM, IgG, IgD and IgE), with IgM representing the initial response. The release of IgG represents the recovery from an infection and IgG protects the individual against reinfection. Mucosal immunity is evaluated by the salivary immunoglobulin that is easily reported in response to exercise. Thus, trained female rowers have a higher salivary IgA concentration compared to non-athletes, yet this elevated IgA level is not affected by a bout of rowing and it is not high enough to protect against upper respiratory tract infections. IgD exists in low plasma concentrations but no immunologic function of this immunoglobulin has yet been identified. IgE also exists in low plasma concentrations compared to IgA, IgM and IgG, but becomes elevated in response to infections brought about by parasites or worms and in patients with immunodeficiency. IgE also becomes elevated in response to allergic reactions and binds to receptors on mast cells and basophilic granulocytes.

Repeated exercise

With the idea that exercise-induced lymphocytosis reflects activation of lymphocytes, it has been evaluated whether the activation becomes even more intense in response to repeated bouts of exercise. Also, it might be that post-exercise suppression of the immune system would become more intense after two or more bouts of exercise. After three bouts of 6-min all-out ergometer rowing, the concentration of lymphocytes becomes higher at the end of the second and third bout compared to the response to the first bout of rowing (Fig. 5.1). Even higher levels were noted on the following day when three additional bouts were performed. Equally important, a lowered concentration of lymphocytes in blood was not observed in the recovery period after the sixth bout. Such observations indicate that the immune system remains alert during a regatta for which two or three races per day may be needed in order to accomplish both heats and finals or because of a requirement to participate in two or several separate events.

The acute response of the immune system, even to repeated bouts of rowing, does not explain why

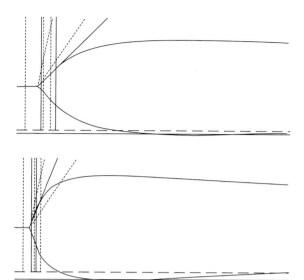

Fig. 5.2 Thrombelastographic presentation of the ability to form a clot in whole blood before and during ergometer rowing (M. Zaar and P.I. Johansson).

rowers are vulnerable to upper airway infections following training. More likely, such adverse events are explained by the repeated exposure to an often wet and cold environment.

Besides the sympathetic nervous system, and more specifically epinephrine, which is important for mobilizing the immune system during exercise, adrenaline is of importance for coagulation. The ability of whole blood to coagulate and to maintain the clot that is formed can be illustrated by thrombelastography. With that system the resistance to rotate a pin in the whole blood sample is evaluated. When the pin is rotated, it takes some time before the clot starts to form but clot formation then proceeds rapidly (Fig. 5.2).

Normally, and as illustrated in Fig. 5.2, the developed clot is maintained, but in some diseased states or in response to medical treatment the clot may be dissolved. Relevant to rowing is that the time to clot formation decreases during ergometer rowing and, furthermore, clot formation becomes faster. Both of these effects can be ascribed to the fact that the function of the thrombocytes is enhanced by adrenaline.

Hormonal regulation in overtraining

Endogenous hormones are important for energy supply during exercise as well as during the subsequent regeneration period. Also, hormonal changes seem to have an essential role in the pathogenesis of overtraining. In this context, testosterone and cortisol are important for protein and carbohydrate metabolism. Changes in blood concentrations of testosterone and cortisol during exercise indicate an alteration of the anabolic–catabolic balance. The ratio between testosterone and cortisol decreases with intensity and duration of exercise and during periods of intense training, or repetitive competitions, and can be reversed by regenerative measures. However, it seems that the testosterone:cortisol ratio indicates the actual physiologic strain in training rather than a case of overtraining syndrome.

In support of a hormonal dysregulation as the mechanism of overtraining, a long-term study revealed attenuated levels of pituitary hormones and cortisol following maximal exercise in the overtraining compared with the normal state. At present, however, the practical usefulness of blood measurements of sexual hormones for diagnosing overtraining remains uncertain.

The sympatho-adrenergic system may also be involved in the pathogenesis of overtraining. Overtraining manifests as a disturbed autonomic regulation, which in its parasympathicotonic form shows a diminished maximal secretion of stress hormones combined with impaired mobilization of anaerobic lactic reserves. This leads to decreased maximal blood lactate concentrations and impaired maximal performance.

Ergometric testing in overtraining

The few existing assessments of the limit of physical performance in the overtrained state indicate speed endurance, or short-term endurance, is impaired and anaerobic lactic capacity is limited. Thus, longer lasting exhaustive exercises are helpful tests for the assessment of overtraining in endurance trained athletes. In this context, exercise duration during overtraining is significantly reduced in comparison to the rower's normal state while the anaerobic alactic performance seems not to be affected.

Although the lactate–performance curve represents a useful tool in the monitoring of training, it may also lead to wrong conclusions. In an example of an overtrained Olympic rower, the maximal lactate concentration during a rowing competition and the corresponding performance were clearly decreased compared to his usual values. The same could be simulated in a 6-min all-out test on the rowing ergometer. However, in submaximal exercise the lactate–performance relationship as well as the corresponding calculation of anaerobic thresholds remained unchanged, which is typical in the overtraining syndrome. The simple orientation on such thresholds would overestimate the actual exercise tolerance.

Assessment of overtraining

No accurate means are available either to predict the onset or detect if failure to adapt has already occurred. It is often difficult to differentiate between what may be abnormal physiologic responses related to a failure to adapt or simply normal responses to heavy training. However, based on the limited research and the many observations by coaches and athletes over the years, the following seem the most promising of possible measurements.

Measurements used previously:
1 Resting heart rate and chronic increases in blood pressure
2 Cardiac arrhythmias (changes in heart rhythm)
3 Increase in white blood cells; increase in eosinophil levels
4 Increase in cortisol levels
5 Chronic hypoglycemia
6 Decrease in muscular power and $\dot{V}O_{2max}$
7 Decrease in muscle glycogen
8 Decreases in testosterone (male) and estradiol (female) or disturbances in free testosterone and bound testosterone; decrease in free testosterone : cortisol ratio
9 Increased lactic acid for standard submaximal exercise

Measurements that may have potential worth:
1 Body composition; abnormal decreases in body fat and lean body mass (LBM) and change in fat : LBM ratio
2 Chronic elevation in core temperature
3 Abnormal liver function tests
4 Changes in endorphin levels
5 Decreases in hemoglobin; chronic anemia ("athlete's anemia"); disturbances in erythropoietin
6 Volume of rapid eye movement (REM) sleep
7 Chronic decrease in blood volume
8 Chronic elevation of skeletal muscle enzymes

The most attractive factors for possible investigation are blood volume, body composition, muscle enzymes, core temperature and red blood cell status, most of which are closely linked physiologically. Periodic submaximal ergometer testing may prove beneficial. Athletes should be tested frequently during periods of high intensity or high volume training using rowing ergometry and work outputs ranging from 60–80% of maximum. Measurements of submaximal heart rate, $\dot{V}O_{2max}$, lactic acid, O_2 deficit and O_2 debt may be useful in predicting and detecting failing adaptation. A test based on three consecutive submaximal efforts on a rowing ergometer, where heart rate and lactate responses during and following 60, 70 and 80% of mean maximal output are measured, has been developed by Hagerman. It is important to conduct most of these measurements during resting or recovery conditions without the immediate effects of previous exercise as examination of possible failing adaptation factors could be masked by the acute effects of a training session.

Altered mood profile

In daily training sessions, the assessment of psychologic profiles may be helpful for the estimation of the exercise tolerance in athletes. This requires clinical experience in closely monitoring athletes. The psychologic profile (e.g., parameters of mood profiling such as strain, deficiency and recovery) as well as ratings of perceived exertion during standardized exercise are significantly disturbed during overtraining in comparison to the normal state. In all cases, the diagnosis of overtraining remains a clinical assessment and requires that organic illness as an underlying cause is excluded.

Prevention and treatment of overtraining

Because it is difficult to identify any clear preliminary or early warning signs of failing adaptation, it is equally difficult to prevent it. Carefully designed recovery periods are as important as the intensity of the specific workout, or series of workouts, in the determination of overall training intensity. As the length of recovery is often overlooked, the insertion of a longer than planned rest, or recovery period, at a critical time in the long duration, or intense, phase of training, may prevent overtraining.

Although some of the measurements discussed earlier may aid in helping to predict or reveal failing adaptation, the most effective measure is the coach's knowledge of the athlete and the self-awareness of the athlete. Not only should coaches and athletes record such daily entries in training diaries as distances, stroke rates, times, total volume, number of hard strokes, heart rates, lactates, etc. but, more importantly, both coach and athlete should carefully and immediately after each training session record their subjective feelings about the workout; this procedure should also be used for major training phases or periods.

Although the cause of failing adaptation is most likely a combination of some or all of the factors discussed, the intensity, speed or rate of training are more critical stressors than the volume of training. Many coaches believe that overtraining symptoms can be reduced or eliminated by a few days of light training when it would be best for the athlete to rest completely for 2–3 days, followed by 3–4 days of easy cross-training. Prevention is preferable to having to cure failing adaptation. In order to minimize the risk of failing adaptation, a periodic training program alternating easy, moderate and hard training periods should be used. One or two days of intense training should be followed by an equal number or more of easy training days. This principle should also apply to weekly planning and 1–2 weeks of hard training should be followed by a week of easy work.

In summary, there is only a subtle difference between the normal responses to heavy training and the abnormal responses associated with failing adaptation, in fact, so finite that it may not be possible to accurately measure, detect and prevent.

Recommended reading

Hagerman, F.C. (1992) Failing to adapt to training. *FISA Coach* 3, 1–4.

Hagerman, F.C., Hikida, R.S., Staron, R.S., Sherman, W.M. & Costill, D.L. (1984) Muscle damage in marathon runners. *The Physician and Sportsmedicine* 12, 39–48.

Kuipers, H. & Keizer H.A. (1988) Overtraining in elite athletes. *Sports Medicine* 6, 79–92.

Nielsen, H.B. (2003) Lymphocyte responses to maximal exercise. A physiologic perspective. *Sports Medicine* 33, 853–867.

Kreider, R.B., Fry, A.C. & O'Toole, M. (1998) *Overtraining in Sport*. Human Kinetics, Champaign, IL.

Urhausen, A. (1995) The overtraining syndrome: a diagnostic challenge. *FISA Coach* 6, 1–4.

Wilmore, J.H. & Costill D.L. (1988) *Training for Sport and Activity, the Physiological Basis of the Conditioning Process*. Wm. C. Brown Publishers, Dubuque, IA.

Chapter 6
Psychology

S.L. Dupcak

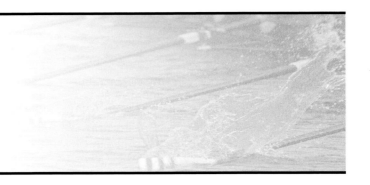

Introduction

In sports, the psychologic component of training and competing is just as important as the physiologic component, and rowing is no exception. Rowers, coxswains and coaches must prepare themselves mentally, as well as physically, in order to meet the ever-increasing standards and achievements in rowing. This chapter addresses the psychologic aspects of racing. Rowing is often called "the ultimate team sport." A rower's heaven is when everyone in the boat is at full power, swinging in perfect unison with one mind and body. Thus, it is crucial to prepare mentally for success as an individual within the boat, as well as a team.

A cornerstone to sport psychology is the phrase, "As we think of ourselves, so we are." The mind is like a mirror that holds the pictures, ideas, thoughts and words we have about ourselves. An athlete's self-image shapes how he or she functions and performs.

The mind has compelling control over the body. For a long time, it was thought to be impossible to run a 4-minute mile. However, Roger Bannister believed he could, and he did. After boldly breaking the 4-minute mile barrier and shattering a long standing "truth," many runners soon joined Bannister at this new performance level. Were they suddenly that much more physically fit? No, but the psychologic paradigm of what was possible changed, demonstrating the power of imagined barriers. This holds true for rowing or ergometer time standards as well. Every year there is a new standard, one which was thought to be unattainable 5 years ago.

Just as a rower learns and repeatedly practices the mechanics of rowing, mental skills must also be learned and practiced. Sport psychology focuses on learning the mental aspects of peak performance by helping athletes understand how their emotions, thoughts, beliefs and attitudes influence their performance. Moreover, developing solid psychologic skills helps rowers effectively deal with the stresses of balancing the multiple tasks of life, while enjoying the thrill and exhilaration of rowing.

Regardless of the level of training and competition over a few years, most athletes and crews are making a similar physical investment. So what determines which crew will get to the finish line first? Many factors, but a much overlooked element involves mental preparation, good coaching, confidence in abilities (as an individual and as a boat) and mental toughness. Positive thinking, confidence, consistency and quality rowing are what will help a team to reach the finish line first.

This chapter focuses on some of the key principles of sport psychology, such as the role of arousal, stress and relaxation on performance. This is followed by a brief discussion of confidence, positive thinking and concentration. The chapter finishes with preparation for competition. This is an introduction and brief overview of some of the sport psychology principles that effect performance. Additional sport psychology techniques such as visualization, effective goal setting, communication and teamwork are equally as important.

Arousal and relaxation

It seems as though stress is everywhere! The pressure to perform well, to make the seat you want or to lose that last pound before race day all impose stress. Not to mention the stresses that come with deadlines at work or school and just trying to keep up in today's fast-paced world. Stress and anxiety are very adaptive emotions that serve to inform us of problems both in the environment and within ourselves. Think of stress as the body's alarm system. The body signals when it is physically or emotionally overwhelmed. The signal is designed to say slow down, make a change, or STOP!

Evolutionarily speaking, stress is an important feedback system and source of information. However, over time, with the increasing pressures faced in the modern world, we have learned to overlook and ignore our bodies' internal distress alarm system. In some circumstances this is not necessarily bad. For instance, many people perform better when they are under a *moderate* amount of stress, but when we are not in control of the stress, it has a significant detrimental impact on physical performance as well as on emotional well-being.

Arousal can be thought of as the psychologic and physical activity of the mind and body. Research in anxiety and stress management shows that athletic performance is maximized when there is an optimal level of emotional arousal. Many experienced athletes have learned to identify the proper recipe of emotions and physical preparation that lead to their best performances. Almost all athletes have experienced at least one poor performance as a result of excessively high levels of anxiety or arousal. Conversely, physical performance also suffers when a rower is not aroused enough.

The best way to assess an individual's peak arousal level is to have him or her reflect upon previous race situations. With races in which the athlete did not meet his expectations, was he flat (underaroused)? Was she overanxious or stressed? What was his level of arousal and anxiety during his best performances? Rowers should try rating themselves on an arousal scale from 1 to 10 for each of their recent races. Notice the patterns that begin to emerge.

A large component of an individual's arousal level is stress and anxiety. Anxiety can take the form of worry ("I don't know if I can make it through the entire race at this pace"). Anxiety can also be manifested physically in terms of butterflies, sweaty palms, feeling fatigued, racing heartbeat, etc. Anxiety is strictly an internal process. It does not exist outside of your head. Certain *situations* may tend to create anxiety (e.g., an important chemistry exam, seat racing, a deadline at work or an important race), but one is not required to become anxious in these situations. People are anxious, situations are not. Anxiety results from interpreting a situation as overwhelming or becoming overly concerned with the outcome or consequences of an event. Thus, anxiety is manageable if the athlete controls his or her thoughts about a given situation. For example, focusing on the outcome of a race (winning or losing) creates tremendous anxiety and arousal, as opposed to focusing on the step-by-step execution of the race plan; thereby keeping arousal to a level at which it helps performance.

Each athlete has his or her own optimal level of arousal. However, it is easy to become under- or overaroused. The typical signs of underarousal include feeling flat, bored or unfocused. Conversely, hyperactivity, an inability to block out irrelevant sensory information, the physical jitters and racing thoughts are signs of overarousal. Athletes must find the level of arousal at which they perform their best. Once that optimal arousal level is found, a rower can use relaxation strategies to calm down or "psyching up" techniques to move toward and maintain your optimal level of arousal, and therefore optimal performance (Fig. 6.1).

Before detailing some relaxation techniques, it is important to understand how and why excessive anxiety and arousal causes deterioration in performance. Anxiety often manifests itself in muscle tension. Thus, the shoulders get tight, legs feel like lead or rubber bands, and arms feel heavy with increased anxiety. Not only does this muscle tension interfere with a rower's physical ability to get up to full slide, lift his or her hands to the catch, or feather effectively, but excessive muscle tension makes the moves very mechanical. With increased anxiety or arousal, and therefore increased muscle tension, rowing technique is compromised and a rower feels

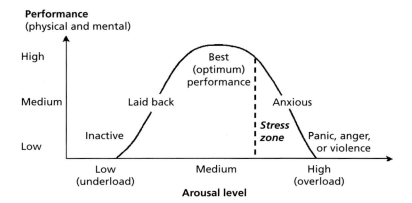

Fig. 6.1 The relationship between arousal and performance.

tired much faster. With anxiety and muscle tension there is no flow, no swing and no powerful movement through the water.

Anxiety also manifests itself in the form of worry. Negative thoughts or worry about one's performance can be overwhelming. This type of anxiety prevents rowers from thinking clearly about what must be done in order to row well. Excessive anxiety is especially dangerous for coxswains, as their decision-making abilities and steering are adversely affected by stress and worry. Furthermore, an overly anxious coxswain can project that worried tone to the crew and make any existing anxiety even worse.

In his book, *Assault on Lake Casitas*, Brad Lewis nicely captured the importance of relaxation in rowing.

> "The stroke is divided into two complementary segments, the drive and the recovery…The drive is all muscle, strength, eye-popping effort. The recovery is cool, subtle, a chance to take a deep breath and prepare for the next drive."

Remember that excessive tension and worry exhaust a rower both physically and mentally at a rate far greater than when he or she is relaxed while rowing. Of course, it is much easier to stay relaxed and breathe on the recovery when you are rowing at 16 strokes·min⁻¹ versus 38 strokes·min⁻¹. A relaxed recovery provides a chance to recuperate and regroup so that you can push even harder on the next drive.

This discussion about relaxation may call forward images of lying on a beach without a care in the world. Yes, this is one form of relaxation, but rowing would be quite challenging in such a relaxed state. Again, there is an optimal level of arousal and muscle tension that enables optimal performances. Some rowers need to be more relaxed to perform their best, while others need to be more physiologically aroused. Fortunately, there are a number of methods that athletes can use to bring themselves to their optimal level of arousal in each performance.

The following is a brief outline of several different coping strategies used to reduce stress. These strategies may be used alone or paired together (e.g., deep breathing and imagery) to facilitate relaxation. Because everyone is different, what works for one person may not be the best method of relaxation for another.

Deep breathing

This is a good relaxation skill that can be used anywhere, at any time and in only a few seconds. Inhale deeply through the nose over a count of three to four. Hold the breath for approximately 2 s, and release it slowly through the mouth, letting everything in the body go loose. Repeat this two to three times. Some people find it useful to say a cue word such as "relax" or "let go" when they exhale.

Progressive muscle relaxation

Progressive muscle relaxation is a simple technique, although it requires practice to achieve maximum benefit. The technique involves the progressive tensing and relaxing of various muscle groups. Begin with your feet and move up to your head, using different muscle groups. For instance, your feet, calves, quads, stomach and back, forearms and hands, biceps, shoulders, neck and, finally, forehead. With each muscle group, tense the muscle, hold the tension for 7–10 s (concentrating on the feeling of the tension) and release, taking a deep breath and noticing the relaxed state. Repeat each muscle group twice before going on to the next muscle group.

Meditation

Meditation is the relaxation of the mind first, followed by the body. It does not necessarily involve sitting in a cross-legged position for hours while humming. There are many different forms of meditation. One of the simplest versions of this relaxation skill is to find a quiet area and begin by focusing on breathing. Deep breaths are not necessary but it is important to pay attention to the airflow in and out. The task is to concentrate on your breathing. As you notice that your mind has drifted, make a mental note of where you went and gently bring your awareness back to your breathing. The goal is to clear the mind of distracting, stress provoking thoughts. Start with 5–10 min·day^{-1}, gradually moving up to longer periods of time.

Visualization

Think about a relaxing scene, such as the beach at sunset, a secluded island or a favorite childhood spot. During moments of stress, imagery can be used to escape to this place and relax. Begin with two to three deep breaths. As you visualize, picture the relaxing scene in as much detail as possible. Note the colors, sounds and even the smells. Immersing yourself in a relaxing scene is calming and enjoyable.

Music

This is a popular form of relaxation and stress management. It can also be used to bring your level of arousal up if you are too flat. You can easily combine music with the imagery (both visualizing the rowing stroke or the race plan, as well as visualizing your relaxing scene).

Many of these techniques require practice before they are effective in reducing anxiety. Each technique should be practiced on a daily basis. After a short period a rower will be more proficient and reap the benefits while performing at his or her optimal level of arousal.

Concentration and focus

The best performances in athletics often occur when an athlete is completely connected in mind and body. It is often referred to as rowing on "autopilot." This is when a rower lets his or her body lead, rowing without any interferences of the mind—a state called "flow." Flow feels effortless, even though the rower is pushing hard. Flow is a state of mind or focus in which a rower is completely connected both mentally and physically with the oar(s), the water and other rowers in the boat. Achieving this flow state feels as if the body has just taken over and it is doing exactly what it has been trained it to do with very little effort. Rowers repeatedly state that they know they are pushing themselves to their limits, but it feels effortless—"everything just clicks." In order to achieve the flow state, a rower must trust his or her body to do what it has been trained to do without forcing the body motions as he or she becomes tired or more anxious.

Concentration busters

Unfortunately, most athletes struggle to achieve this state of "flow" or complete concentration and connection. There are many things that get in the way and ultimately disrupt a rower's focus. The primary concentration buster is worry. Worry about what you can do; worry about what you cannot do; worry about the competition; worry about the race conditions, etc. These worries guarantee a disruption in focus and concentration not only in practice, but most certainly during races.

Another problem for many rowers is focusing on factors that are outside of one's control. These include distractions such as the competition, weather, water conditions, a bad warm-up and previous race mistakes. There is very little that can be changed, if anything at all, about these factors so there is no benefit to thinking or worrying about them. These thoughts are guaranteed to disrupt your concentration and prevent you from achieving the flow state.

Focusing on past or future events are other common concentration busters. Thinking about past events includes finish positions in previous races, mistakes, and feelings following a loss or poor performance. Mistakes and loss occur in every rower's career. While we can learn from the past, dwelling on the mistakes simply creates tension, interrupts focus and ultimately disrupts flow.

The same can be said for focusing on future events. These are the "what-ifs." "What if I am down in the first 500 m?" "What if I lose the race?" "What if I catch a crab?" Worrying about what could happen breaks concentration on the present situation (what you are doing at that moment), increases muscles tension and leads to poor performances.

Improving concentration and focus

In order to improve concentration and chances of achieving "flow," there are a number of things athletes can do. First, practice with distractions present. Try to recreate the racing situation as much as possible, purposely adding distracters in order to gain experience ignoring the distractions and letting the body take over.

Second, use cue words, which are quick reminder words for what a rower should be focusing on during a practice or race. These are usually techniques oriented words such as: "drive" for leg drive, "quick and smooth" for the finish, or "swing back" for the rhythm of the back swing. The idea is to maintain the rower's focus on what he or she is doing at that moment — not what just happened (or happened earlier in the race or in previous races) and not what needs to happen later in the race. With the exception of a general race plan, it does little good to worry about what needs to happen later in a race, as it pulls focus off the task at hand and away from the flow state.

The third method of improving your concentration is to practice non-judgmental thinking. Try to avoid evaluating performances as "good" or "bad." Mistakes should not be ignored, but look at the performance as it is. There are always positive and negative things about a race or practice. Again, choose one or two mistakes to focus on in the coming weeks of practice and let everything else go.

Fourth, establish a race or practice routine. Doing basically the same routine of physical and mental preparation for each race will help structure your time before and during races. Also, routines bring about comfort. At a time when you are feeling most nervous, you need the comfort of falling into a routine.

Fifth, practice eye control. Avoid letting your eyes wander to irrelevant cues during races. There is no reason to focus on the other rowers or spectators if it is anxiety provoking. Keep your focus on your own boat, your race plan and what you need to do to make this a good race for you.

Finally, focus on the present by concentrating on the job at hand. I call this "staying in the moment." In focusing on the here and now, or what you are doing at that moment, you are able to block out distractions. This includes thinking about previous mistakes or worries about what is to come. For example, it does little good to think about the power twenty you will take in the third 500 m when you are sitting at the start. This only leaves you open to thoughts of the pain that you will feel in the third 500 m, or "what ifs" such as, "What if I am down by a boat length?"

Being completely focused and achieving the "flow state" is not easy. Just like anything else, it takes practice and time. You can begin by challenging yourself to stay focused for 10 min at a time in practices. Initially you might alternate 10 min of full concentration followed by 10 min of regular focus (whatever you currently think about in practice). Gradually, you can lengthen your time of focused practice and racing, thereby getting closer to achieving your flow.

The power of positive thinking

One of the factors that often disrupt our focus is negative thinking. The way a rower thinks about or interprets an event has a direct correlation on how

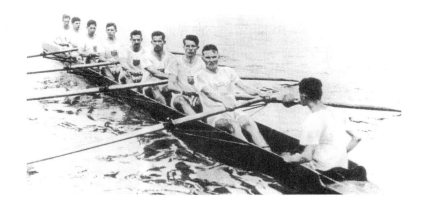

Fig. 6.2 The American eight winning the 1924 Olympic championship.

he or she performs in that situation. In other words, if a rower goes to practice thinking, "I really don't want to sit in that boat for 2 h in 37°C weather," then his practice most certainly will not be fully productive or effective.

Our behavior is a product of our thoughts. Perhaps you are familiar with the "battle of the voices" in your mind. That is, one voice is saying, "Yes, I can do this," while the other voice is saying, "No, I can't—I can't push that hard." These two voices seemingly get louder during hard practices and on race day. Doubting one's self is normal, especially when rowing at very high stroke rates while trying not to rush the slide, and realizing that you are a boat length behind and your legs are screaming with exhaustion. Although this is challenging, the ability to overcome fears, believe in one's self and think positively is what separates the champions from the rest of the crews.

Confidence and positive thinking

The power of positive thinking is remarkable, and it is a skill from which everyone can benefit. Self-confidence provides the building blocks or the foundation of a positive attitude and positive thinking. Self-confidence is built from a number of factors including one's general belief in one's self and past experiences. It is a belief system that says, "I can" and "I will," as opposed to, "This will never work" or "I can't." Having confidence in one's self as a rower is believing in your abilities in any situation, regardless of whether you are in front of or behind the competition, rowing through 2 ft waves, or on a virtual sheet of glass. "I know I can" is a very differ-

ent statement than "I think I can." And the performances are undeniably different.

This is called "true confidence." It is the ability to believe in yourself and your performance in any given situation. It is not a false belief, but realistic to your present ability level. True confidence is always with you. It understands the natural highs and lows of practice and racing. True confidence can pull a rower out of a slump, or realistically help a rower evaluate the performance of a lifetime.

Believing in your abilities to succeed is vitally important in both practice and competition. However, you must also be realistic. In other words, to always believe that you will win a race is sometimes unrealistic, as some crews or rowers are just faster than others for reasons beyond your control. Having confidence in yourself does not always mean winning the race, but rather prevailing through all conditions to reach your goals and succeed. Confidence is built through practice, previous experiences and hard work. These, in turn, require a daily commitment to positive thoughts in order to build your self-confidence (Fig. 6.2).

Controlling your negative thoughts

Fortunately, controlling negative thoughts is not as difficult as it may seem. The first step in controlling negative thoughts is recognizing them. When warming up for practice or a race, you may find yourself thinking, "I feel tired" or "I don't feel ready today." These thoughts are detrimental to performance. Negative thinking is the equivalent of having a coach, coxswain or teammate constantly making negative comments, such as, "You can't do this. You will never be as fast as the competition. Your stroke is all wrong." Just as a rower would not voluntarily stay with such a caustic coach, it is equally as caustic and detrimental to have these negative thoughts running through his or her mind! Recognizing the negative thinking patterns and turning them around into positive thoughts is vital to successful performance.

Race day jitters are an excellent example of how negative thinking can adversely affect performance. Epinephrine (adrenaline), which is significantly increased on race days, can have the effect of making one's body feel heavy or tired. These feelings are commonly misinterpreted by the mind as, "I am tired" or "I feel so heavy and tight." Athletes often fail to recognize that they are just nervous, a normal and physiologically desirable reaction. Without a moderately increased level of epinephrine, the body may not achieve the great things that happen in competition. Thus, athletes need to recognize the physiologic signs of increased epinephrine, interpret them correctly as nervousness, and appropriately deal with that nervous energy by warming up extremely well and using relaxation techniques. Now the negative thoughts of, "I'm so tired. I am not ready," are turned around to, "Okay, I am prepared, excited and ready to go. What I am feeling is normal and natural. It's my body's way of saying, 'I'm ready!'"

Blocking the negative thoughts is not always easy. Having scripted and prepared positive thoughts is the most effective way to remain in control of the mind. Begin by keeping a brief record of "typical" negative thoughts encountered during practices and on race day. Next, develop some positive statements to say to yourself (sometimes repeatedly) in order to turn the negative pattern around.

Being a positive thinker does not mean that a rower never has negative thoughts. It is unrealistic to think that an athlete would always be confident. Furthermore, stress and anxiety tend to enhance negative thoughts and make that little voice in your head even louder. Once a rower acknowledges that it is completely normal to feel nervous, scared or anxious before a big race, he or she can frame these feelings in a positive manner such that they will not interfere with success.

Turning off your negative thoughts

There are a number of different strategies for "turning off" negative thoughts. Each will work differently for different people. A survey carried out on sources of stress in champion athletes identified a number of strategies for positive thinking. In order to maintain their motivation, champion athletes stay focused on the goals and the things that are going well. Another successful strategy is to surround one's self with reminders that trigger positive thoughts by posting positive thoughts or quotes onto your mirror, steering wheel, foot-stretchers or even the rower in front of you. Positive athletes have often adopted a "watch me do it" attitude when they are challenged. Successful athletes also frequently remind themselves that they are well trained and prepared for this race, competition or challenge. Strong rowers understand that there is an appropriate time to question one's self, but in general, especially at races, just do what has been done in practice and concentrate on doing it better. Finally, many successful athletes use some variation of the "thought stopping" technique.

An important and highly useful technique for managing negative self-talk is "thought stopping." Thought stopping is just what the name implies. You catch yourself in a destructive negative thought pattern and signal yourself internally to stop in some manner. This signal could be the image of a stop sign or someone waving a red flag. You could yell, "STOP!" to yourself, snap your fingers or gently snap a rubber band on your wrist. Once you have stopped the negative thought, replace it with a more constructive thought.

For example, first you recognize a negative thought. "I am already down four seats off the start!" Signal yourself to internally stop this panicky thought process by imagining a huge red stop sign. Now replace the negative thought with a positive thought, such as, "Okay, I have stopped their movement and I am coming back into them one stroke at a time, one seat at a time."

Developing a positive mindset takes practice, repetition and time. In the beginning, there may be setbacks and negative thinking. Eventually, more of the negative thoughts will be automatically "turned off" or "tuned out" and the rower will notice a difference in his or her attitude, enjoyment and success. Remember, "what the mind believes in, the body will achieve."

Psychologic preparation for successful racing

Because of the natural elements in rowing, there are many things that are not in a rower's direct control on race day. Most experienced rowers have seen the chaos that can occur at races. However, with a little mental preparation and planning, athletes can learn to put these distractions out of their minds, thereby preventing any significant disruption in concentration or performance. The goal is to stay relaxed, comfortable and focused on the days leading up to and including race day. The more centered and controlled an athlete feels, the more likely he or she is to perform up to expectations and ability level. Thus, preparing for race day includes not only the physical workouts, but also the mental preparation for staying calm, controlled and confident in any situation that could arise on race day.

Mental race preparation gives a rower an edge up on the competition. The confidence gained from being prepared and knowing that nothing is a surprise will benefit a rower and crew all the way down the course. In order to feel confident and controlled on race day, athletes need to follow the "three P's":
1 Plan purposefully
2 Proceed with a positive attitude
3 Pursue persistently
These are inherent aspects of mental planning for successful racing.

Elements of a successful race — mental preparation

There are three critical aspects of mental race preparation and planning for success. The first component is the pre-race plan. This includes both the physical and psychologic aspects of the warm-up. The second component of mental preparation is the race focus plan. This includes the physical race plan, a race focus plan and motivational words that help rowers sustain speed, power and control through-

out the race. The third component is the refocus plan which is designed to help rowers "expect the unexpected."

Pre-race plan

Many rowers follow the same or a similar pre-race warm-up every time they launch for a race. It is also beneficial to do a similar psychologic warm-up. This might include making realistic, positive self-statements (e.g., "We are well prepared for this race;" "I know I can do this!") and visualizing the many scenarios that can occur within a race plan (e.g., a slow start, being up at the 1000 m, feeling spent at the 1500 m, and being down by two seats in the last 20 strokes). When a rower, or crew, has a well-defined and practiced pre-race plan, even the most nerve-wracking, stressful and important races seem more normal and achievable.

Imagery is an important part of pre-race mental preparation. Imagery or visualization prepares an athlete for all situations, thereby removing any element of surprise during a race. Surprises cause excessive anxiety. Anxiety causes increased muscle tension, an inability to concentrate, negative thinking and frantic ineffective racing. With the use of imagery, rowers can remain calm and controlled regardless of whether they are ahead or behind. Some rowers may be hesitant to imagine themselves behind in a race. It is important that you not dwell on the negative, but instead have an exact plan for coming from behind and be prepared if the situation should arise. Imagery and a pre-race plan are important aspects of executing a race the way you want. It brings the element of control into your performance, in a situation where you actually have very little control of the others around you, the water, the weather or the race officials.

To make a pre-race plan, think back to your most successful races and try to determine how and why you were successful. What did you physically do to prepare? What thoughts were going through your mind? How did you feel (e.g., excited, really nervous, calm and controlled, etc.)? You can also do this exercise for the races that went poorly. Over time, you should start to see a pattern with what works well for you both physically and mentally in your race preparation. Write down the physical and

Table 6.1 Example pre-race plan.

Home/hotel	Boathouse	Launch/warm-up	Stake boats
Physical preparation			
In bed early	Check rigging	Shove off; boat is one	Remove last layer of clothes
Good meal	Coach/boat meeting	Stern 4/bow 4 warm-up	
Boat meeting	Check cox-box battery	2 power 20s	Check oarlocks
Shower to loosen and wake-up	Stretch, be warm	High 10 settle 20	Stretch to relieve tension
	Last minute, water-condition check	10 minutes before race, do start sequence	
		Power 10s	
Mental preparation			
Go over race plan and each move	RELAX with deep breaths	If warm-up wasn't good, remember that's what it's for	Close eyes; image start sequence
Image race with conditions	Excitement level up; remember I love this		3 deep breaths
		If tight, relax shoulders I can do this!	I am ready for this! GO FOR IT!
		Confidence; believe in me Be Positive!	

psychologic actions in the days and hours leading up to the very start of the race (Table 6.1). As you draw upon the thoughts and procedures that served you best in the past, write down your physical preparatory actions, including such things as stretching, checking the oarlocks and making sure the cox-box works. Also, write down your general psychologic warm-up including mental imagery of the race plan, positive self-statements and relaxation techniques. Writing this down provides a concrete plan to evaluate and refine if necessary, as well as helping you and your crew maintain consistency in your race preparation.

Race focus plan

The second component of race preparation is the race focus plan. As a rower, you demand so much from yourself physically that it is critical to develop a strategy for pushing beyond your limits psychologically. Aside from the general physical race plan (e.g., the starting sequence, your power moves, the sprint sequence), a psychologic race plan includes general cues and reminders for each part in the race that is difficult. Self-statements such as, "Lengthen out," "Relax and breathe," "I can do this" and

"Power in the water" should be part of your focus plan just like your power moves. As you plan out a race, identify the areas of the race where you need these positive self-statements. These powerful and succinct reminders are called cue words. To create your own set of cue words, think of the statements that best motivate you. Using technique oriented cue words such as, "Hands up at the catch" are also an extremely important part of the race plan, as rowing technique tends to deteriorate with exhaustion. Cue words, stated or thought forcefully with emotion and conviction can override the physical pain and allow you to dig deep within yourself, calling upon your reserves.

Committing to your prepared mental race plan (which corresponds to each segment of the physical race plan) will help immensely when the legs are burning in the middle of the third 500 m. Energizing cue words such as, "GO!"; "Push it NOW!"; or "POWER!" can be useful, as well as the following thoughts: "Don't give up an inch"; "We have trained too hard to let it slip away"; "No regrets"; "It's now or never." Regardless of how we look at it, racing hurts. Thus, it is vitally important to develop a mental focus plan to get through the pain, push past our limits, and succeed!

Race refocus plan

The third aspect of planning for success is "expecting the unexpected." No matter how well prepared for a race, there are bound to be some organizational or weather-related hassles that are beyond control. Thus, it is also important to have a refocusing plan, or a plan of action to help put the hassles out of your mind and focus on the task at hand—executing the race plan. The refocus plan is designed not only to help you get back on track when something goes awry, but also to stay focused and calm in all situations. Ultimately, a rower's anxiety and muscle tension remain in control, such that racing is productive, efficient and successful.

To develop a refocusing plan, think about situations in which there were unwanted distractions. Also, reflect upon the times that you could have benefited from regaining emotional or physical control quickly. For each situation, outline a strategy (with your coach and crew members) that will help you refocus and overcome the problem. The following are some situations to develop refocusing plans: pre-event hassles (e.g., late bus, mix up at registration, etc.); poor weather conditions; false starts; poor start; catching a crab; poor performance in the first 1000 m; etc.). This is a "what-if" list. "What if I am down in the first 500 m of the race?" "What if I cannot get a full warm-up in?" With a refocus plan, rowers can actually plan out a strategy or response for each of the scenarios. There is a corresponding element of comfort (and therefore reduced level of anxiety) knowing that there is a plan in place and should one of the "what-ifs" actually occur, you know exactly what to do.

The refocus strategy should include an action plan, some cue words and positive self-statements. The key to successful refocusing plans is *practice*! You and your crew have to simulate these situations and practice using your refocusing plans, in order to feel confident that you can handle anything.

Once you have established a pre-race plan and a race plan that you feel confident in, following the race plan becomes extremely important. If the plan is executed to the best of your ability, then there is little else you and your crew can do. You cannot control what the other boats do; you can only control what your boat does and what you do

personally. Furthermore, racing success involves staying focused on each section of the race. A common mistake made by many rowers is to focus on the outcome of the race (who wins). Instead, you need to concentrate on executing the race plan one step at a time and doing it to the best of your ability. The outcome will be decided based on this. Why waste mental energy stressing about the outcome of a race or the competition when the only thing you can control is your own performance? Remember, rowing ability does not change from one event to the next. However, the situation and racing conditions will change. Be prepared.

Conclusions

Successful performances in rowing are not completely a matter of chance, but rather a choice. This choice is hidden in how you talk to yourself, how you feel about yourself, and what you expect from yourself and your crew. Mental preparation involves training and practice just as the physical preparation is necessary for racing success. There are several aspects of mental training and sport psychology, including many that have not been discussed in this chapter. A key to mental training and rowing success is maintaining a calm, controlled and confident mindset. Positive thinking, focused concentration and following a planned race strategy are essential aspects of reaching your rowing potential. You have the capacity to choose how you feel, think and focus. Choose to feel and think positively. Perform as you choose to perform. We are a product of what we repeatedly do and feel. Excellence is not an act, but a habit.

Recommended reading

Bennett, J.G. & Pravitz, J.E. (1987) The profile of a winner: Advanced mental training for athletes. *Sport Science International*. Lansing, NY.
Csikszentmihalyi, M. (1990) *Flow: The Psychology of Optimal Experience*. Harper & Row, New York.
Horn, T.S. (1992) Advances in sport psychology. Human Kinetics Publishers, Champaign, IL.

Loehr, J.E. (1994) *The New Toughness Training for Sports: Mental, emotional, and physical conditioning from one of the world's premier sports psychologists.* Plume/Penquin Putnam, Inc., New York, NY.

Martens, R. (1987) *Coaches Guide to Sport Psychology.* Human Kinetics Publishers, Champaign, IL.

Nideffer, R.M. (1992) *Psyched to Win.* Human Kinetics Publishers, Champaign, IL.

Orlick, T. (1987) *In Pursuit of Excellence.* Coaching Association of Canada, Ottawa.

Porter, K. (2003) *The Mental Athlete.* Human Kinetics Publishers, Champaign, IL.

Chapter 7
Training

Z.B. Babraj and S. Volianitis

Introduction

Training describes the capacity of the human body to adapt to increased demands brought about by structural and functional changes specific to the applied workload. The load is a stimulus that, while being applied, causes fatigue. If the load is significant and not over-stressful, fatigue is followed by a recovery, which not only restores the energy level but also creates "supercompensation" (Fig. 7.1).

Supercompensation is a delayed effect of the response to a given load manifested by the synthesis of protein, restoration of fuel storages and increases in hormonal and enzyme activities. If supercompensation is not followed by another workload within a short time, it disappears. The consequences of a given workload are not only related to the specificity of that load (i.e., the type of exercise chosen), but also to the volume and its intensity.

The immediate effects of training are crucial for selecting the right intensity (strength of application and frequency), volume (mileage, time or number of repetitions) and the method used. The character and extent of the immediate training effect determines the overall structure of training cycles and the order of different individual exercises in the training session. For example, small changes in the intensity of exercise, or improperly chosen recovery periods in interval workouts, challenge different metabolic capacities than those planned. Scheduling exercises without considering the effects of previous training sessions may create an undesired reaction in the body. For instance, the effect of anaerobic exercise with lactate acid accumulation will be intensified if preceded by speed exercises. On the other hand, if anaerobic exercise follows long distance aerobic work, the effect is reduced.

Long-term adaptation in rowing is based on the cumulative effect of many training sessions. To reach a cumulative effect, each training load is executed when the effects of previous sessions are still present. On the other hand, if recovery is extended between workouts the effects of the previous training session are lost. In that situation the best possible result is maintenance of the training status. For optimum performance athletes must start each workout during the recovery phase from a previous workout, before full recovery and supercompensation is reached. Waiting for the complete delayed effect to take place is only beneficial in the peaking cycle before important competitions, but is not desired in the gradual progressive training process. The controlling elements for the planning of training are frequency and the rest time between training sessions. After executing several training sessions with incomplete recovery, it is advisable to add a rest session to allow the body to rebuild and improve capacity for exercise (Fig. 7.2).

Progressive load

To improve performance, the athlete follows a training process of systematically and gradually raised loads, which periodically creates an overload. Workload in training is increased in accordance with each individual's physiologic and psychologic ability and his or her rate of improvement or adaptation. The principle of progressive increased load is the basis for planning of training from the microcycle to the multiyear cycle. This principle applies to the programs of all athletes, regardless of age or ability. A progressive load refers not only to the volume and intensity, but also to the quality and ratio between general, basic and specialized types of work.

One mistake made by athletes and coaches is the use of repetitive loads. When planning a training program, a constant workload leads to dissipation of the training effect and eventually to physical and psychologic deterioration causing a decrease in performance capacity. A set routine day after day becomes boring and after some initial progress causes a plateau in athletic performance, and if continued long enough eventually leads to a regression in results. This applies to repetition of the same

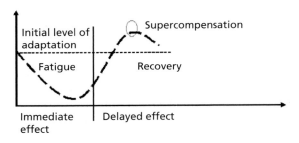

Fig. 7.1 Training effects of a single workout with an optimum load.

workout as well as to the same type of load applied in bigger cycles (Fig. 7.3).

This does not mean that the loads must be changed all the time. Some functions require repetition of the same type of load to achieve improvement. During the training process various exercises, abilities and body functions have different rates of improvement. Substantial improvements in flexibility can be achieved in a few weeks, while significant progress in aerobic capacity takes months to years. Stepwise increases also differ significantly. In order to keep improving, flexibility must be varied every 2–3 days, strength weekly and endurance monthly. The increase or change in training load should also be governed by the rate of improvement in performance.

For different characteristics such as endurance, speed and strength, the proper length of each step or progression and the amount of increase in load is different. Also, each individual's speed of adaptation is different. For improvement in technique the increase in load may come from raising the difficulty of exercises, introduction of new technical skills, change of the rhythm or in rigging. The time or the number of hours spent training is important. Annual raises of 20–30% in training volume are not uncommon in early stages of development but, as an athlete matures, the increase becomes smaller. Once an athlete reaches the elite level, further increases of load through raising the volume of workout time is seldom an option. In order to ensure progressive development in adaptation and performance, there must be a careful manipulation of volume, intensity and frequency of different types

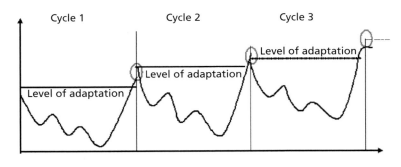

Fig. 7.2 Cumulative effect of multiple training sessions.

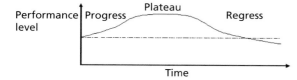

Fig. 7.3 Effect of applying a constant workload on performance.

of loads. An athlete's physical development stage, psychologic profile and ultimate goal within a specific timetable will influence the rate of change or increase in workload.

Multilateral development

A well-organized training system builds on multilateral development but that does not mean random cross-training of different sports. For young athletes multilateral development means development of motor skills and physiologic abilities in a sequential order relative to age for proper periodization of each stage of development. In developed athletes, multilateral development is expressed through general work executed in the transition and preparatory phases.

A good strength training program includes an introductory multilateral development phase. This serves not only to develop strength in all major muscle groups, but also to secure the development of small muscles in addition to the strengthening of connective tissue and the training of the nervous system. Strength training also improves anaerobic metabolism, develops flexibility and coordination, and indirectly improves speed, agility, reaction time and intramuscular coordination. Without strength training the athlete will face eventual performance-related problems and even injury. A lack of coordination may lead to limitations in learning and improving weightlifting techniques. Underdevelopment of the connective tissue, antagonistic and stabilizing muscles makes performance-related muscles less effective and eventually leads to injury.

Championship performance tests a body to its limits, involving abilities, systems and reserves that cannot be developed using only the specific training process. Preparing the body for future specialization is a way of laying the groundwork for future success. Multilateral development integrates both physiologic and psychologic processes which, in the execution of complex tasks involved in sport, are interdependent. For this reason, general development of all body functions and multiple motor skill development with psychologic shaping are crucial to perform effectively at a high level.

Specialization

Specialization has two unique and seemingly contradicting aspects to it. The first aspect is complexity, which explains why an athlete must develop all abilities needed for the final performance. Even elite rowers, in order to improve, must perform much of their training using exercises and methods that do not seem related to rowing performance including development of general strength, endurance, speed, flexibility and coordination. Also, while rowing, or using the rowing ergometer, much time is spent at intensities and rates much lower than those used during racing.

The second aspect is specificity, which requires extensive training specific to rowing. Rowers need a good general development in all physical capacities to be successful. However, at a certain point an athlete can overbuild general characteristics so that they become an obstacle to high-level performance. For instance, strength is important for rowers but excess general strength development decreases a rower's efficiency by the development of muscle mass that is not directly involved in rowing but is carried and supplied with oxygen. Also, an overbuilt body will have higher muscle tension and that influences technical ability in the boat.

Individualization

Each athlete has to be treated individually according to his or her ability, potential and learning pattern. The individual effort capacity and work adaptation depends on factors such as biologic age, experience, training and health, rate of recovery, body somatotype and gender.

The key to individualization in rowing is control of the load and testing. Systematic testing allows for the development of a profile of the athlete's weaknesses and strengths, which help the design of a more accurate individualized training program and the monitoring of specific loads and their effects.

In rowing, individualization is simple for a single sculler but becomes more challenging with participation in bigger boats. Crews may consist of rowers who can move the boat together but have very different responses to a given training program. For example, during a workout aimed at the anaerobic threshold (AT) some of the rowers may be working at lower intensity, while others work at AT level and some above that. In order to ensure that all athletes are developing their AT, the following workout can be individualized by using smaller boats such as pairs or singles.

It is important when programming any activity not to get entrapped by "institutionalized truths" based on statistics and standardized programs. Every rower should, ideally, develop his or her own specific way based on his or her individual characteristics. For example, there are successful rowers who train 600 h·year^{-1} while others train 1500 h.

Variety

Elite athletes spend as much time at their sport as high-level executive professionals spend at work. The volume and intensity of the workouts are increasing, and exercises are repeated over and over again and elite rowers often train more than 1000 h·year^{-1}. With such an amount of work there may be a problem in distinguishing between overtraining and mental fatigue. Whereas overload (easily mistaken for overtraining) is required for performance improvement, mental fatigue, which has its roots in boredom and monotony, is not. When building short- and long-term programs, it is important to pay attention to the impact variation can have on the result.

Periodization of the annual training process into weekly, monthly and seasonal cycles provides variety in the program and prevents staleness or boredom. When planning individual training sessions, various methods can be used to keep each session stimulating and thus attractive. Keeping variety in the training process has the benefit of not only preventing monotony, but, more importantly, of speeding up progress through active participation. Variety maintains the athlete's attention and stimulates the central nervous system keeping the athlete alert and magnifying the effect of the workouts.

After many years of training, even with adequate periodization, there are only a few things that can be varied. Sometimes radical changes of environment and activities for even a short period can help. The transition period, or early preparatory stage, is well planned for different activities, to get away or to learn new skills. Such changes of practice are also included in the beginning of the final preparation up to a main event.

Active participation

If an athlete becomes bored or stale, the worst thing he or she can do is to do nothing. Active participation, also called mental engagement, is the cornerstone of development. Progress, especially in the form of permanent change, is achieved through full engagement of the senses. It is essential that the athlete is not only involved with, but also excited about the venture he or she has embarked upon. The passive presence of an athlete who simply follows a routine leads the way to underachievement and attenuates permanent progress. Likewise, a coach who simply executes a given program, without engaging in the commitment to its outcome, will derail even the best athlete. Without focus on an objective and a commitment to execute each step properly, neither athlete nor coach can guarantee any progress, regardless of the number of hours spent training.

Active participation is the daily input of psychologic energy into the training and competition process. Through the continual integration of psychologic and physical energy, the body and mind become programmed to perform and physiologic development is directly influenced by active participation in the process.

The way an athlete, especially a young or developing athlete, is introduced to the training process is fundamental to his or her development of mental aspects of dealing with performance. Overestimating talent or potential is accompanied by setting excessively high performance goals. This inevitably leads to frustration, anxiety, loss of confidence and underachievement. On the other hand, underestimating or ignoring talent leads to setting excessively low performance goals and leads to sloppiness or boredom in the training process and thereby underachievement.

Types of training

Endurance

Endurance represents the ability to maintain certain exercise intensity over a given time. Endurance is relative to factors such as intensity (e.g., speed, force, load, tension), technical efficiency, muscle adaptation and the athlete's psychologic state during execution of the work. The different types of endurance are determined by intensity and duration of the effort. A 2000 m rowing race is a medium-duration event, influenced by both aerobic and anaerobic capacity, with approximately 70–80% of energy supplied aerobically.

Aerobic capacity

Aerobic capacity training must develop both the transportation of oxygen and the utilization of oxygen by the muscles. The two main factors determining performance in rowing events are maximal oxygen uptake ($\dot{V}O_{2max}$) and muscle adaptation. The primary factors affecting an athlete's average speed in a rowing race are $\dot{V}O_{2max}$ and his or her technique, which is an important determinant of the economy of movement, defined as the energy cost for a given speed. How long a given speed can be maintained is also dependent on efficiency in fuel utilization.

While $\dot{V}O_{2max}$ may be the best expression of aerobic capacity, the AT provides the most accurate starting point for monitoring and designing endurance training for rowers. The AT is the point where the balance between production and removal of lactate cannot be maintained and accumulation of lactate in the blood stream begins. The most accurate way to measure AT is by blood sampling (e.g., from a fingertip or an earlobe) during an incremental workload test on a rowing ergometer from very low to maximum intensity efforts. Yet, results obtained on a rowing ergometer may not be representative of rowing on the water. For elite athletes testing in the boat is ideal. This test allows the coach to identify the AT as the minimum intensity that will produce a training effect. AT is usually identified at a lactate concentration around $4\,mmol \cdot L^{-1}$.

$\dot{V}O_{2max}$ is probably the most reliable measure of aerobic capacity and expresses the rower's endurance potential. However, AT shows how much of this potential is used by a rower. A well-developed rower shows very little fluctuation in $\dot{V}O_{2max}$ values during the annual training cycle while his or her AT varies greatly, as AT is sensitive to changes in the quality (intensity, duration and frequency) of the training load.

Training near the AT level improves aerobic capacity the most, while at the same time it reduces the risk and occurrence of overtraining. Training close to AT also prepares the rower for the maintenance of a higher training intensity without the accumulation of blood lactate. Also, training above the AT level causes a loss of aerobic capacity. In fact, if training is more than 10% above AT level it does not bring much more progress and may be detrimental to endurance.

Improvement of aerobic capacity can also be achieved at lower intensity than AT, but then longer duration is required. Structural changes leading to improvement of oxygen utilization at the muscular level are best produced through low intensity, long duration workouts. This is important because reducing the work intensity is not only desirable for many young athletes, but also for elite rowers trying to reduce the risk of overtraining and injury.

Up to 90% of the work in the preparatory phase of the annual training cycle and approximately 70% of the work during the racing season is performed below $2\,mmol\cdot L^{-1}$ of lactate concentration. In the annual program 90% of rowers workload should be under the AT level ($4\,mmol\cdot L^{-1}$ lactate concentration). For those loads below a lactate concentration of $2\,mmol\cdot L^{-1}$ to be effective, they must be applied in the form of long duration workouts (1–2 h). Such low intensity, long duration loads involving fat metabolism are important for development of aerobic metabolism and rowing technique. If such a base is not developed, the rower will not be able to carry out more work at the AT level and his or her recovery time will be longer.

While the training load eliciting a lactate concentration below $2\,mmol\cdot L^{-1}$ can be carried out daily, the workouts near or at AT level ($3–4\,mmol\cdot L^{-1}$) have their limits. Training at the AT level brings results quite fast but, if not controlled, can compromise the development of the aerobic base. The suggested frequency for a workout at AT is up to two times per week in the preseason period and one time per week during the racing period.

Improvement in the AT allows the rowers to train more and with higher quality at race speed. The best intensities for improvement of average race speed are loads at 90–98% of $\dot{V}O_{2max}$ or at $5–8\,mmol\cdot L^{-1}$ of blood lactate concentration. For the improvement of $\dot{V}O_{2max}$ three to five workouts per week are sufficient.

Anaerobic capacity

$\dot{V}O_{2max}$ versus the rowing technique determines the average race speed. However, it is the anaerobic capacity that can improve an athlete's chances to win a specific race. A rowing race over a 2000 m course demands high intensity with a power that leads to a lactate concentration above $30\,mmol\cdot L^{-1}$. This exceeds the intensity level at which a rower reaches $\dot{V}O_{2max}$ ($\sim 10\,mmol\cdot L^{-1}$). Although there is no precise determination of how much anaerobic metabolism contributes to the outcome of a rowing race, the estimation from ergometer testing suggests that up to one-third of the energy comes from anaerobic energy systems.

Improvement of anaerobic capacity can be achieved primarily in two ways:
1 Increase in the rate of glycolysis, which means an increase in the rate of lactic acid production
2 Improvement in lactate tolerance

It is often the sprint at the end of a race that determines its outcome. At the end of the race there is no need to conserve energy and the speed of the boat will be decided by the stroke rate and force. Therefore, the effectiveness of the sprint will be decided by how fast the rower can release energy from glycogen which means also how rapidly lactic acid can be produced.

Lactate tolerance training is focused on improving muscle buffering capacity. As an improvement in AT allows the athlete to row at higher speeds without accumulating more lactate, so will an increase in the muscles' buffering capacity enable the rower to work at a higher intensity before severe acidosis occurs.

At the start of the race, energy is derived from a chemical compound (creatine phosphate). However, there is only enough creatine phosphate to supply energy for 5–10 s. Training at maximal intensity improves rowing power by transferring the strength acquired in weight training into explosive high rate stroke power. Improvement at maximal intensity will increase the rower's speed and technique, especially at the start.

Endurance includes the ability to tolerate fatigue and the discomforts that come with it. For this reason, the importance of psychologic preparation to deal with monotony, pain and motivation is essential. The ability to perform great amounts of work over long periods of time as needed to develop all aspects of endurance is critical for success in endurance sports (Table 7.1).

Strength

Rowing presents the unique challenge of trying to balance high development of the physiologic abilities of endurance and strength. The expression of strength is force (mass × acceleration). Increases in force can come from raising both mass and acceleration, or by raising either mass or acceleration independently. Because of the different ways in which maximum force is produced and the specificity of sports, strength has many expressions. The most general methods used in evaluating strength are absolute and relative strength.

Maximum strength refers to the maximum force exerted in one attempt and does not take into account body weight. *Relative strength* represents

Table 7.1 Categories of training intensities.

Level	Objective	Lactate (mmol·L^{-1})	Intensity level (% of 2 k max)	Heart rate (% of max HR)	Duration (min)	Duration/rest Single stimulus
I	Regeneration, fat utilization, capillarization, basic endurance, technique	<2	65–70	65–75	30–150	30–150 min Rest: none
II	Development and stabilization of basic aerobic endurance, technique —economy	1.6–3	70–80	75–85	30–120	30–120 min Rest: none
III	Anaerobic threshold improvement, aerobic capacity, oxygen uptake, glycogen storage exchange	3–5	80–85	85–95	20–60	45 s–30 min Rest: 15 s–10 min
IV	Transportation, maximal oxygen uptake, speed endurance	5–8	85–95	95–100	15–45	1–10 min Rest: 1–10 min
V	Racing, race modeling, speed endurance, lactate tolerance, maximal oxygen uptake, tactical abilities, technique economy	8–18	95–100	Max	6–20	1–7 min Rest: 2–15 min
VI (a)	Anaerobic capacity Lactic: lactate tolerance, start and sprint abilities technique—high rate coordination	>10	Max	Max	3–12	40 s–2 min Rest: 1–5 min
(b)	Non-lactic: speed, power	<3	110	Not relevant	2–6	5–20 s Rest: 1–3 min

the ratio between an athlete's absolute strength and body weight. In rowing, relative strength is more important to performance than absolute strength.

Another way to categorize strength in practical training is to express the general and specific strength. *General strength* refers to the strength of the whole body and is the foundation of the strength program development, regardless of the sport. General strength must be highly developed during the first few years of training for beginners and also be a part of training for all levels of athletes during the preparatory period. *Specific strength* is the strength of the muscles particular to the rowing motion which includes characteristics such as speed, acceleration and resistance. The specific strength must be developed to the maximum possible level toward the end of the preparatory phase and maintained throughout the season for all elite class athletes. It is not essential for young, developing or beginner athletes to spend a substantial amount of time developing specific strength because rowing and the rowing ergometer provide enough stimuli to increase specific strength. Also, specific strength training should not be undertaken until

the correct rowing technique is developed. In rowing, specific strength should be developed simultaneously with muscular endurance.

Strength is commonly substituted, or interchanged, with the word power. *Power* is a product of speed and strength and it relates to the ability to perform the maximum force in the shortest period of time. In rowing, power is not a major factor but it has an influence at the start and at the initiation of a sprint when there is need for rapid acceleration of the boat by increasing the pressure on the water and the stroke rate.

Rowers should not do all their strength training in the weight room. Circuit training, ergometer and water rowing with added resistance should account for the majority of the strength work. It is only fair to mention that there are still questions raised as to whether general power strength training with weights has an influence on performance of the elite rowers. However, there is little doubt about the positive influence of general strength development on overall fitness and in injury prevention.

Strength improvement not only has an influence on speed and power, but also provides the basis for strength endurance. The ability to perform high power application over a long period of time or distance (such as a 2000 m rowing race) is *strength endurance*. Because there are approximately 220–250 strokes in the rowing race the average strength impulse can only be a fraction of the maximum power it is possible to deliver in one stroke.

While the need for strength training in rowing is unquestionable, the best way to develop strength is still a matter of discussion. The two major issues that influence this discussion are related to overbuilding muscles to the point of impeding aerobic utilization capacity of the muscle on the one hand and disturbing intramuscular coordination by raising tension in the antagonist muscles in the rowing motion on the other. Rowers need balanced development to avoid injury; however, too much tension in the opposing muscles can decrease the speed and strength of the agonist muscles' contraction. This is visible especially at the catch where premature tension may cause a significant negative force and during the drive where a lack of relaxation in the antagonist muscles decreases the effectiveness of the stroke and brings early fatigue.

Strength training

Maximum strength improvement comes from three ways of adaptation:
1 *Muscle enlargement:* growth of the cross-section of the muscle (proliferation of contractile material — myofibril).
2 *Improvement of nerve–muscle connection* through shortening time of recruitment of motor units, increasing firing rate and engagement of a greater number of muscle fibers in a shorter period of time.
3 *Improvement of intramuscular coordination* between agonists, antagonists and synergists muscles during movement (tension–relaxation).

Training to improve recruitment of more fibers in a shorter time does not lead to enlargement of muscle mass. The growth of the muscle is the result of intensification of tension development. Following intense strength training the body overbuilds protein (supercompensation) resulting in muscle mass growth. The effectiveness of this process

decreases when the intensity is close to maximum or during aerobic efforts. That is why lightweight rowers who want to increase maximum strength without gaining weight should use very high loads (over 85% of max) with few repetitions to avoid overbuilding muscle mass.

Strength training methods

The major methods of strength development training are the following:
1 *Maximal loads:* maximum strength development with minimal muscle enlargement and great improvement in the tone of the muscle. A load of 85–100% of the strength capacity is used in a short maximum effort (1–6 repetitions) with slow execution of motion.
2 *Body building or muscle enlargement:* characterized by a large number of sets of repetitions with a submaximal load of 60–80%. The execution of the movement is rapid to slow and ends with complete muscular failure. There are several variations of this method:
• low number of sets leading to complete failure at the end of every set
• higher number of sets leading to complete failure only in the last set
• every set and number of sets performed to complete failure
The athlete starts with a load allowing for the execution of 8–10 repetitions. After a few weeks the load is increased, or the recovery between each set is decreased and/or the number of sets increased to maintain progress.
3 *Circuit training* combines improvement of strength, speed and endurance. Circuit training is used for general development. It is also used as a warm up before the main strength training and in the preparatory cycle. The circuit should consist of a minimum of 8–12 exercises. The choice of exercises depends on the goal of the session. The load may be varied 30–60% of max or body weight. Exercise should be performed fast. Circuit training stations can be organized by number of repetitions or by time (30–60 s on each station) with a short rest time between stations.
4 *Muscular endurance training* is similar to circuit training with resistance varying 40–60%. The

number of repetitions is 30–80 or more per set. The speed of the work is slow to medium. Muscle endurance is the basic method used for maintaining strength for athletes in endurance sports. An excellent way to develop general strength is through the use of free weights. Training with free weights or dumbbells is demanding for the body and should only be used with the correct technique. Maximum strength development workouts are most effective when the athlete is rested. In the competition period, specific strength workouts should be limited to one, maximum two sessions per week with simultaneous decrease in volume and increase in intensity over the period.

Strength development phases

Like other characteristics of sports abilities, strength development has a cyclic profile. There are three stages of strength development:

1 *Multilateral development:* general strength development of the entire body without specific development for a particular sport

2 *Direct development:* strength development in a group of muscles that are specific to rowing

3 *Specific development:* strength development with simultaneous modeling of speed, endurance and rowing technique

Periodization is done not only at different levels of long-term development, but also repeated throughout every yearly cycle (Fig. 7.4).

Within the annual cycle, the goals for strength training vary depending on the time of the year. In the first part of the preparatory period athletes should aim to reach the level of strength from the previous year. During the second part of the preparatory period they should strive to improve chosen parameters of strength. During the competition season they should maintain the level of strength from the preparatory period. And finally, during the transition they should prevent major losses of strength.

Planning and periodization

The need for periodization is found in the principles of the training process. Analyzing the training process by using periodical tests and performance results we can see three distinguished phases

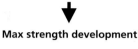

General

(Mobility, flexibility and connective tissue development)

Max strength development

Transformation to sport specificity

Development of muscular endurance and power

Maintenance of max strength

Fig. 7.4 Phases of strength development.

involved in reaching a high level of adaptation: *development, stability* and *periodical loss of high level adaptation.*

These three natural phases of building, reaching and losing high level performance adaptation are the premises for cycles of the training process. For the best overall development of the athlete, annual periodization should be a reflection of long-term periodization. Periodization should divide the program into smaller cycles, allowing better control over the training process which aims at peak performance for the main competition of the year. The length and specific content of each cycle depend on the stage of long-term development.

For athletes who are trying to peak for Olympic performances, which come only every 4 years, each year between the Olympic Games should have a different profile with an emphasis on building or improving specific and varied characteristics.

Traditionally, annual periodization includes three major cycles: *preparatory*—with general and preseason subphases, *racing* and *transition.*

Preparatory cycle

Accumulation is devoted to the development or rebuilding (for high level athletes) of general abilities. Accumulation should be the longest phase of annual periodization and, depending on the stage of development, can take 40–60% of the yearly cycle. Accumulation is the foundation of the annual pyramid where the top is final performance. The quality of the upcoming competitive season and peaking is directly related to this period.

Intensification (preseason or specialized subphase of the preparatory period) aims to lay the foundation for maximum and above maximum level loads used in the next phase of training. This phase is a progressive step from accumulation level loads to more specific and higher intensity but still submaximal loads. Exercises used in the intensification phase are rowing specific. This phase takes 20–25% of the annual cycle and may purposely cut into the beginning of a racing season. In this case competitions are programmed into training and performed with a strategy reflecting training tasks for this period.

Racing cycle

Transformation is the most important task of training during the racing season to transform the high level of athletic shape formed during the preparation stage into the best possible performance in a specific competition. Training during the transformation phase has maximum and above maximum intensity loads separated by low intensity loads to secure recovery. Transformation also includes a few workouts aimed at maintaining basic development with an overall decrease in volume. All work should directly simulate racing conditions or aim at modeling a desired performance.

If training is well-planned, *peaking* can produce a 2–6% improvement of the regular season performance, depending on the level of the athlete. Peaking is usually used in the period between the regular racing season and the main event (e.g., World Championships or Olympic Games). Peaking cycles may take 2–8 weeks.

If peaking is done well after a short period of time (1–2 weeks) the athlete can drop almost immediately to an average level of physical conditioning. Peak performance cannot be held for prolonged periods. The training that brings peak performance is based on the sequence:

Max load→breakdown→rebuilding→improvement
(stress)   (damage)   (repair)

This sequence can actually cause more damage than is needed but, because of the accumulation and intensification training, the body can cope with this challenge for a limited time. During this time results dramatically improve, but eventually, if excessive damage accumulates, central fatigue may develop as a mechanism that prevents irreparable body damage.

Transition cycle

The main target of the transition cycle is to remove the physical and mental fatigue accumulated during the competitive phase and to regenerate stores for the accumulation phase. During this period of approximately 2–6 weeks of active rest, a change of environment and fun recreational type activities are recommended. The transition period is crucial to secure long-term adaptations. A timely and efficiently planned transition allows the athletes to start a new cycle on a higher level of basic athletic shape which can lead to a higher development level for next year's peaking. A break that is too long and/or passive between the racing season and the next preparatory cycle leads to detraining (Fig. 7.5).

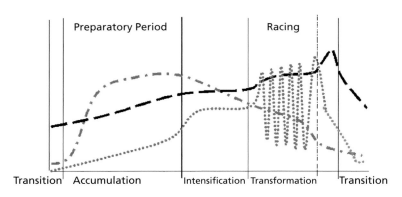

Fig. 7.5 Example of yearly periodization. Bars, performance level; dots, intensity level; bars and dots, volume of training.

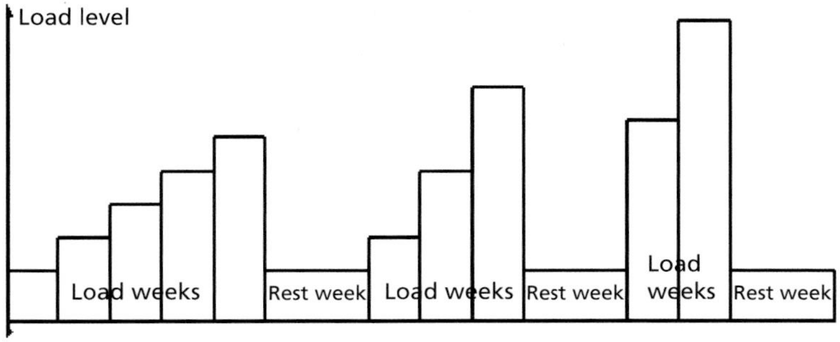

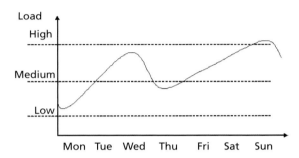

Fig. 7.6 Example of load rhythm application.

Fig. 7.7 Example of a weekly microcycle with a variation of high, medium and low level loads.

Load and rest

Even carefully planned increases in the training load may lead to stress. To avoid overtraining, the increase in the load versus the recovery period is applied rhythmically (Fig. 7.6).

To balance the load–recovery relationship, training periods are divided into smaller cycles including 2–6 microcycles. The microcycle lasts usually a week and may take on different forms such as developmental, modeling, regeneration. Depending on the training period, several microcycles of increased load are followed by a week of significantly reduced volume. The ratio between build-up and recovery microcycles can be 5:1 to 3:1 in the preparatory period, and 2:1 to 1:1 in the racing period (Fig. 7.7).

The design of the individual microcycle should accommodate the rhythmical application of the load. One week's schedule should consist of variation of high, medium and low level of loads.

Recommended reading

Astrand, P.-O., Rodahl, K., Dahl, H.A. & Stromme, S.B. (2003) *Textbook of Work Physiology: Physiological Bases of Exercise*. Human Kinetics, Champaign, IL.

Bompa, T.O. & Carrera, M. (2005) *Periodization Training for Sports*. Human Kinetics, Champaign, IL.

Fritsch, W. (2000) *Rowing: Training–Fitness–Leisure*. Meyer & Meyer Sport, Oxford, UK.

Herberger, E., Beyer, G., Harre, D., Kruger, H.-O., Querg, H. & Sieler, G. (1977) *Rudern*. Sportverlag Berlin, German Democratic Republic.

Korner, T. & Schwanitz, P. (1985) *Rudern*. Sportverlag Berlin, German Democratic Republic.

Maglischo, E. (1982) *Swimming Faster: A Comprehensive Guide to the Science of Swimming*. Mayfield Publishing Co., Palo Alto, CA.

Matwiejew, L.P. (1979) Structure of sports training. *Sport Wyczynowy* **12**, 13–24.

Nolte, V. (2005) *Rowing Faster*. Human Kinetics, Champaign, IL.

Chapter 8
Performance assessment

K. Jensen

Physical testing in rowing

Physical tests evaluate performance, which in rowing is the shortest time for a 2000 m distance. The result is influenced by factors such as direction and speed of wind, waves and current. Furthermore, there may be a need to evaluate the individual work capacity in a boat including as many as eight rowers. Conversely, physical performance tests reveal the strengths and weaknesses of the individual athlete's physiologic profile and may thereby guide adjustments to the training program. Also, assessment of physical performance can be useful for selection of the team.

Physical assessment evaluates both physiologic and biomechanical factors related to rowing performance based on work capacity, body dimensions and rigging. Figure 8.1 shows different phases of a rowing stroke during 6 min all-out rowing ergometry incorporating physiologic and biomechanical measures.

On a rowing ergometer, efficiency describes the relation between the energy used and the work performed but the validity of this measurement for rowing on the water, where a more complex technique determines the translation of external work into boat speed, is questioned. The use of the "sliding" rowing ergometer for the determination of the metabolic cost provides a better approximation and improves the validity of such calculations. A stationary rowing ergometer is fixed on the floor and the rower moves back and forth whereas a sliding ergometer is placed on wheels that allow the ergometer to move (slide) underneath the rower who has a larger mass compared to the ergometer and thus remains close to the same position (Fig. 8.1). Using such a system approximates the assessment of the combined ability to produce large external work and its translation into boat speed. When two, four or eight ergometers are linked the coordination of the whole crew can be evaluated.

Field testing

Rigging adjustments to the size and the strength of the crew are important but they are left almost exclusively to the experience of the crew and its coach. Only few data are available on how a change in the angle of the oar related to the boat and the gearing (i.e., the relative length of part of the oar inside the oarlock) affects boat speed. Thus, there is a need to determine the inboard distance to the oarlock, the length of the slide on the seat, the length of the oar and the position of the rower and the oar relative to the strength of the rower and the length of his or her arms and legs.

It is well established that timing of the blades in the water is precise among international rowing crews but the profile of the force on the oar and the applied stroke length may be different across boats or even among rowers in the same boat (Fig. 8.2).

Coordination between hands and legs is important both for the application of force on the oar

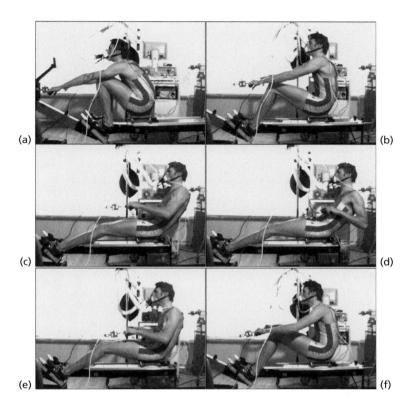

Fig. 8.1 Rowing in an instrumented Concept II ergometer. (a) The start of the drive; (b) first part of the drive; (c) second part of the drive; (d) finish; (e) first part of the recovery; (f) second part of the recovery.

handle and for the timed entrance of the blade into the water. In four heavyweight male rowers from a national team, the movement of the hands and the seat together with the force applied on the handle and the load on the seat were measured during 6 min all-out ergometer rowing. At the beginning of the stroke, the legs move the seat backwards, while the arms remain stretched. Conversely, at the finish of the stroke the legs are fully stretched while the arms are bent. In Fig. 8.3 a large loop of the curve indicates a difference between the start of the movement of the legs and that of the hands. Force on the handle peaks at about 950 N or corresponding to the mass of the rower (96 kg). Accordingly, the load on the seat decreases by ~73% during the stroke to reach its lowest value just before the first half of the drive and increases to 22% above body weight before the end of the stroke. During the first part of the recovery the load on the seat is close to body weight. Accordingly, body weight appears to influence the ability to develop a large force during the stroke.

Crew selection

In order to cover both physiologic and biomechanical aspects of rowing performance assessment, measurements should be both relevant and specific to rowing competitions. Especially for crew selection, the interaction between different rowers of a crew cannot be simulated accurately during laboratory conditions and therefore the final selection is likely to be decided on the water. A common procedure to select rowers for the crew is to perform selection races between boats while switching rowers according to a matrix, a procedure called "seat racing."

Matrix selection

Water trials in smaller boats are one way to select the fastest crew. In Canada and the USA, a matrix process called "seat racing" is used for a clear, fair and open selection. "Seat racing" can last several days and rowers race in various pair combinations a

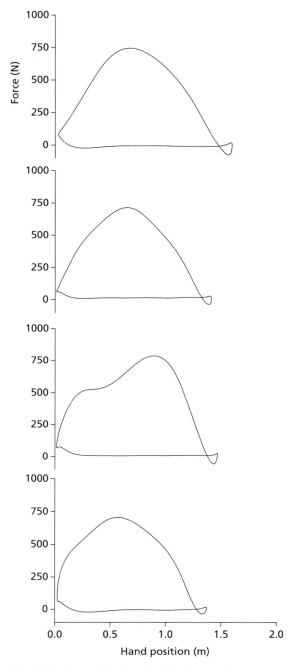

Fig. 8.2 Stroke profiles showing the force on the oar related to oar movement during rowing a coxless four at submaximal level. Zero is the catch position.

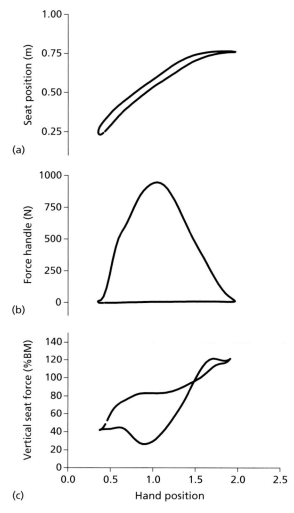

Fig. 8.3 (a) Seat position; (b) handle force; (c) vertical seat force in percentage of body mass (% BM) related to hand position during a 6 min all-out ergometer rowing ($n = 4$).

number of 2000 or 3000 m trials or whatever is considered a valid distance for the competition. The rowing cadence can be predetermined by the coach or left to the choice of the oarsmen. Also, the selection races can be performed side by side or in time trials. Points are awarded according to the placing in the race and a ranking list is developed after each race. An example for five bow side and five stroke side rowers is provided in Table 8.1. First, combinations A are tried for 3–5 days prior to the race; subsequently, in a similar fashion all combinations are tried out.

Laboratory testing

In the laboratory, the rowing ergometer offers the possibility to assess the individual physiologic capacity under standardized conditions. In order to simulate a 2000 m race, performance over 6 min is often used, although most races on the water take longer. At the 2005 World Rowing Championship, the races were won over times that varied between 5:23 and 7:18 min:sec for men and between 5:58 and 8:07 min:sec for women and the estimated ideal time for a world championship regatta is 6:24 (5:34–7:37) min:sec (see Table 1.5). Accordingly, an ergom-

Table 8.1 Combinations of pairs: "A" group including five pair combinations starts the matrix selection, then "B" etc.

Stroke side / Bow side	Tom	Josh	Ed	Bob	Chris
Paul	A5	E5	D5	C5	B5
Mike	B4	A4	E4	D4	C4
John	C3	B3	A3	E3	D3
Beppe	D2	C2	B2	A2	E2
Brian	E1	D1	C1	B1	A1

eter performance over 6 min would be appropriate for the very best rowers only. Alternatively, worldwide competitions and even championships on ergometers are carried out over "2000 m" corresponding to 5:38–6:02 min:sec for men and 6:28–6:57 min:sec for women (Concept II, best results, 2005). As a consequence, rowing would be expected to be an aerobic sport, and rowers are among the athletes with the highest $\dot{V}_{O_{2max}}$. The anaerobic energy system is considered to account for 20–30% of the total energy requirements.

The capacity of the anaerobic energy system increases with muscle mass and rowers try to balance training between aerobic and more intense anaerobic intensities in order to optimize performance. Lightweight rowers are limited by body weight and for these athletes it may be impossible to increase muscle mass and still make weight for competition. Accordingly, lightweight rowers might be more dependent on their aerobic power and capacity than rowers in the open class.

External power during ergometer rowing

As can be derived from the world records for different age groups, the best times for heavyweight men and women correspond to an average external power of 578 and 383 W, respectively, and 472 and 310 W, respectively, for the lightweight class (Fig. 8.4).

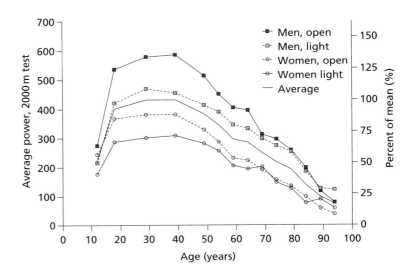

Fig. 8.4 Average power during "2000 m" rowing on a Concept II ergometer. Calculation is based on the world records for different age groups, men, women, lightweights and from the open class.

From 12 to 18 years of age, performance increases from 53% to 93% of the best record or ~7% per year (a steeper increase for men). Conversely, performance decreases gradually from the age of 40 from 99% to only 23% at the age of 90 years or by approximately 1.6% per year (Fig. 8.4). If it is assumed that anaerobic energy contributes to performance ~25–30% and ~20–25% for men and women, respectively, and that work efficiency is ~18%, power for the men and women record holders corresponds to a $\dot{V}O_2$ of 5.9–6.7 and 4.1–4.8 L·min^{-1}, respectively.

Endurance capacity

At a submaximal power, rate heart rate (HR) and blood lactate express the relative intensity of exercise. Following training, lower values of HR and blood lactate indicate that the relative intensity is reduced (i.e., the athlete has increased his or her endurance capacity). Several protocols are used to establish the work intensity that elicits a blood lactate level of 4 mmol·L^{-1}. Most protocols use progressive, submaximal work rates separated by recovery periods allowing time for sampling of blood. Based on the chosen protocol, a lactate and HR profile is established. The profile reflects the endurance capacity and a shift to the right indicates an improvement. However, several factors including diet, training, blood sampling site (artery or vein), lactate analyser, and measurements based on plasma, whole or hemolyzed blood affect the lactate profile. Furthermore, the lactate profile may be influenced by the duration of the work bout, the length of the recovery period and the specific ergometer used.

Maximal aerobic power

An ergometer test with steps of increasing workload can be used to describe endurance when combined with measurements of HR and blood lactate concentration at the end of each step. This progressive test can be used as a rough estimate of $\dot{V}O_{2max}$, as mainly $\dot{V}O_{2max}$ will set the upper limit of how many steps the rower is able to complete before exhaustion. A range of steps applied to a wide range of

fitness levels, body sizes and gender is provided (Table 8.2). From Table 8.2, rowers have to find the level that relates to their fitness level.

The test may include 5–7 continuous steps of 5 min work until exhaustion. The first two steps ~10 min should be with low intensity such as "warming up" and the last step should be a maximal effort. Maximal aerobic power (MAP) is calculated as the power of the last completed step plus the fractional yield from the last, not completed step. A relation exists between MAP and $\dot{V}O_{2max}$ (Fig. 8.5). Accordingly, $\dot{V}O_{2max}$ can be calculated as:

$$\dot{V}O_{2max} \text{ (mL·min}^{-1}) = \text{MAP} \times 13.7 + 287$$

MAP is about 8% lower than the average power of a 2000 m ergometer test, indicating that the anaerobic energy system is more involved during a 2000 m test.

Ergometer tests to evaluate different performance aspects

To evaluate different aspects of performance five tests on a rowing ergometer (100 m, 60 s, 2000 m, 6000 m and 60 min all-out tests) have been proposed to be completed during 1 week of training. From these performances a power–endurance curve can then be constructed and the relation between

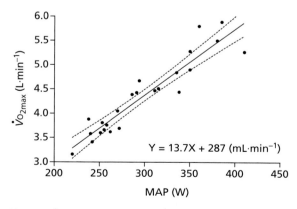

Fig. 8.5 $\dot{V}O_{2max}$ in relation to maximal aerobic power (MAP) calculated from a step test. Included is the linear regression line with its 95% confidence interval.

Table 8.2 Step tests are including a maximum of seven steps (step 1 and 2, "warming up"). Choose one out of 21 levels of fitness. Row for 5 min on each step and not lower than the chosen average W. The result is calculated from the last completed step plus fractional yield coming from the last not completed step.

Step test	Step 1	Step 2	Step 3	Step 4	Step 5	Step 6	Step 7	End pace
Level 1	44	55	66	77	88	99	110	2:27
Level 2	48	60	72	84	96	108	120	2:23
Level 3	52	65	78	91	104	117	130	2:19
Level 4	56	70	84	98	112	126	140	2:16
Level 5	60	75	90	105	120	135	150	2:13
Level 6	64	80	96	112	128	144	160	2:10
Level 7	68	85	102	119	136	153	170	2:07
Level 8	76	95	114	133	152	171	190	2:03
Level 9	84	105	126	147	168	189	210	1:59
Level 10	92	115	138	161	184	207	230	1:55
Level 11	100	125	150	175	200	225	250	1:52
Level 12	108	135	162	189	216	243	270	1:49
Level 13	116	145	174	203	232	261	290	1:46
Level 14	124	155	186	217	248	279	310	1:44
Level 15	136	170	204	238	272	306	340	1:41
Level 16	148	185	222	259	296	333	370	1:38
Level 17	160	200	240	280	320	360	400	1:36
Level 18	172	215	258	301	344	387	430	1:33
Level 19	184	230	276	322	368	414	460	1:31
Level 20	196	245	294	343	392	441	490	1:29
Level 21	208	260	312	364	416	468	520	1:28

Table 8.3 Power in short and longer term tests compared with the 2 km test in (I) Danish National team, (II) Italian, men's team and (III) USA, men's sculling group.

	I (n = 17) (% 2 km)	II (n = 20) (% 2 km)	III (n = 5) (% 2 km)
Anaerobic strength and power tests			
100 m	175 ± 17	174 ± 16	188 ± 16
60 s	154 ± 12	150 ± 8	149 ± 3
Aerobic power and capacity tests			
6 km	84 ± 4		79 ± 2
60 min	74 ± 3		

power obtained in the four tests and that during the 2000 m performance test are used to describe the anaerobic (100 m, 60 s) and aerobic ability (6000 m and 60 min) of the rower.

Successful international rowers could act as a reference for younger and less experienced rowers (Table 8.3). If a rower is within the reference level in the tests for his or her anaerobic power and capacity, but lower in the aerobic capacity tests, it might be a good idea to try to improve endurance. This is the most common situation for younger rowers (Fig. 8.6). Sometimes, young rowers are able to perform well above the reference in a short test while they have great difficulty in completing a 60 min performance test at a reasonable level.

Although performance is different, in absolute terms, between light and heavyweight rowers and between men and woman, no difference is observed between groups of Danish national rowers when power is expressed relatively to the average power in the 2000 m race performance in any of the other four performance tests. Thus, rowers fit the same

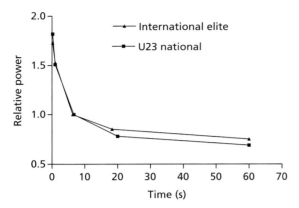

Fig. 8.6 Relative power during 100 m, 60 s, 2 km, 6 km and 60 min of all-out ergometer rowing on a group of U23 ($n = 23$) and international elite rowers ($n = 17$).

equation when it comes to strength and endurance indices. Also, international level rowers seem to fit almost the same equation (Table 8.3) showing current results from groups of rowers from Denmark, Italy and USA, although the US team was slightly more dependent on anaerobic power (personal communication: Lars Christensen, Beppe De Capua and Kris Korzeniowski).

$\dot{V}O_{2max}$

Rowing performance is related to $\dot{V}O_{2max}$ (L·min⁻¹). In order to compare the level of fitness among rowers of different body size, $\dot{V}O_{2max}$ needs to be expressed in units that are scaled to body mass. Because $\dot{V}O_{2max}$ represents a volume uptake over time it scales to "a characteristic" length in the second power ($L^3 \times L^{-1}$) and thereby also roughly to

the body surface area ("the surface law"). Rowers in the open class therefore have higher values than the lightweights (typically ~6.5 vs. ~5.6 L·min⁻¹ for World Class oarsmen). Conversely, when $\dot{V}O_{2max}$ is expressed relative to the body mass, the light rowers have the highest values (75 vs. 68 mL·min⁻¹·kg⁻¹). Therefore, when comparing $\dot{V}O_{2max}$ between rowers with different size, $\dot{V}O_{2max}$ is related to body size with a slightly steeper relationship than expected from the surface law. For a group of 117 rowers, the relationship between $\dot{V}O_{2max}$ and body weight is best described as a 0.73 power function. This expression is independent of body size and is more appropriate when physical fitness is compared between groups of rowers or individuals with different body size. Following such expression of aerobic fitness, rowers rank among endurance sports such as running and cycling. The average $\dot{V}O_{2max}$ for Danish male rowers is 221 mL·min⁻¹·kg⁻⁰·⁷³. For a 100 and 75 kg male rower, this corresponds to a $\dot{V}O_{2max}$ of 6.4 and 5.2 L·min⁻¹, respectively. For female rowers ($n = 32$), $\dot{V}O_{2max}$ is 179 mL·min⁻¹·kg⁻⁰·⁷³. For an 80 and 62 kg female rower this corresponds to $\dot{V}O_{2max}$ of 4.4 and 3.6 L·min⁻¹, respectively.

Recommended reading

Jensen, K. (2005) Monitoring athletes' physiology. In: V. Nolte, ed. *Rowing Faster*. Human Kinetics, Champaign, IL. pp. 25–30.

Jensen, K., Johansen, L. & Secher, N.H. (2001) Influence of body mass on maximal oxygen uptake: effect of sample size. *European Journal of Applied Physiology* **84**, 201–205.

Chapter 9
Nutrition

L. Burke

Introduction

Rowing involves prolonged training sessions that are typical of an endurance sport. By contrast, elite crews and scullers typically take 5–8 min to complete their events over a 2000 m course. International events provide for open ("heavyweight") and lightweight categories of competition. Therefore, while rowers must be strong and powerful, some also need to meet a weight target. With such diversity of characteristics, it is not surprising that nutritional concerns of rowers involve an amalgam of challenges (Table 9.1). This chapter provides a practical overview of strategies to address these issues.

Achieving the ideal physique

The biomechanical requirements of rowing favor athletes with long levers (long limb lengths) and a large muscle mass that is capable of producing high power over a sustained period. Typically, rowers are taller, stronger and heavier than other endurance-trained athletes. Indeed, some studies show an increase in the mean height and lean body mass of elite competitors over the past decades and a difference between competition winners and non-finalists. Although rowers move their own body mass, they are supported by the boat and the buoyancy of water, reducing the energy-cost involved in movement. As a result, although rowers are leaner than their sedentary counterparts, they typically carry higher body fat levels than other endurance-trained athletes (e.g., distance runners and road cyclists). Lightweight rowers are an exception to this, because they need to maximize their effective lean body mass within their weight targets. Although many rowers achieve their ideal racing physique as a result of genetics and training, others need to undertake special dietary programs to achieve their goals.

Nutrition to optimize gains in mass and muscle mass

Gains in size and strength are achieved during the growth periods of adolescence, and in adults as a result of an appropriate resistance training program. Nutrition can have an important role in maximizing net gain in muscle mass, by optimizing the time over a day that is spent with a positive nitrogen balance and minimizing the duration of periods of negative nitrogen balance. Although total protein intake often attracts the most attention of the nutritional issues involved in muscle gain, it is likely that most rowers consume more than enough protein for growth and maximal response to resistance training. Instead, the nutritional factors of most importance are likely to be total energy intake and the timing of nutrient intake in relation to training.

To maximize the outcomes of growth and resistance training, an athlete must consume adequate energy to cover the cost of training as well as the building of muscle protein, itself an energy-expensive process. Strategies to achieve a

Table 9.1 Common nutritional issues arising in rowing.

Physique issues
- Nutrition support to increase muscle mass and strength through specific resistance training program; especially in heavyweight rowers
- Nutrition support to achieve and maintain generally low body fat levels to optimize power to mass relationship; especially in lightweight rowers
- Nutrition support to meet growth needs during adolescence
- "Making weight" — achieving weight targets prior to each race in lightweight rowing; risk of dietary extremism and disordered eating resulting from frustration with weight control

Training issues
- High energy and carbohydrate requirements to meet a heavy training load and growth needs during adolescence or active gain of muscle mass
- Practical difficulties in consuming sufficient energy and carbohydrate intake in a busy day
- Aggressive recovery needed between training sessions (refuelling, rehydration, repair and adaptation)
- Adequate protein intake to meet increased requirements because of heavy training, and to promote gain in muscle mass and strength in response to resistance training
- Adequate fuel and fluid intake during training sessions
- Consideration of ergogenic aids to enhance the response to resistance and interval training: creatine loading

Competition issues
- Preparation of adequate fuel stores for race day: fuelling for multiday regattas and competition meets
- Post-race recovery between events, or between heats, semi-finals and finals
- Consideration of ergogenic aids to benefit race performance: bicarbonate/citrate loading and caffeine supplementation
- Travel: traveling to major competitions and on competition circuit

high energy intake include the planning of frequent meals and snacks across the day. In addition to increasing total energy intake, consuming nutrient-rich snacks before, during and after training sessions provides an opportunity to enhance the acute response to the workout. The intake of relatively modest amounts of high quality protein (10–20 g protein, providing 3–6 mg essential amino acids) after a resistance training session increases net muscle protein balance. There is also some evidence that additional benefits might come from consuming the protein snack *before* the training session, and by adding a carbohydrate food or drink to the mix. Further studies are needed to identify the optimal types, timing and combinations of nutrients consumed as training snacks. However, to meet a range of recovery nutrition goals as well as to contribute to total energy and nutrient needs, the rower should consume meals and snacks supplying carbohydrate and protein in relation to key training sessions (Table 9.2).

Nutrition to reduce weight and body fat levels

At some point in the season or in their careers, many rowers wish to reduce weight and body fat levels. In the case of heavyweight rowers, a desire to achieve a leaner physique is often seen at the beginning of the season when they are returning from a substantial level or period of deconditioning. Indeed, many rowers will achieve a substantial weight loss over the rowing season as a result of their heavy training volume. Although leanness is a characteristic of elite rowers, heavyweight rowers have not typically joined the groups of endurance sports in which athletes seek to minimize their body fat levels, or to achieve levels that are below what seems natural for the individual. However, losing body fat is a particular concern for lightweight rowers who try to manipulate their total body mass and to maximize the muscle:fat (power:weight) ratio of their physique.

There are a number of reliable and valid techniques for physique assessment. These range from techniques that are best suited to the laboratory (e.g., underwater weighing and dual-energy X-ray absorptiometry [DEXA] scans) to protocols that can be undertaken in the field (Fig. 9.1).

In practice, useful information about body composition can be collected from anthropometric data such as measurements of skinfold (subcutaneous) fat, body girths and circumferences (Fig. 9.2).

Coaches or sports scientists who undertake anthropometric assessments on rowers should be

Table 9.2 Carbohydrate-rich choices suitable for special issues in rowing.

Carbohydrate-rich choices for pre-race meals
Breakfast cereal + low-fat milk + fresh/canned fruit
Muffins or crumpets + jam/honey
Pancakes + syrup
Toast + baked beans (note this is a high-fiber choice)
Creamed rice (made with low-fat milk)
Rolls or sandwiches
Fruit salad + low-fat fruit yogurt
Spaghetti with tomato or low-fat sauce
Baked potatoes with low-fat filling
Fruit smoothie (low-fat milk + fruit + yogurt/ice cream)
Liquid meal supplement

Carbohydrate-rich foods suitable for intake during training (50 g carbohydrate portions)
600–800 mL sports drink
2 × sachets sports gel
1–1.5 sports bars
2 cereal bars or granola bars
2 bananas
60 g jelly confectionery
450 mL cola drinks

Recovery snacks — to be eaten post-exercise, or pre-exercise in the case of resistance training to promote refuelling and protein responses
(Each serve provides 50 g carbohydrate and at least 10 g protein)
250–350 mL liquid meal supplement or milk shake/fruit smoothie
500 mL flavored low-fat milk
Sports bar + 200 mL sports drink
60 g (1.5–2 cups) breakfast cereal with 1/2 cup milk
1 round of sandwiches with cheese/meat/chicken filling, and 1 large piece of fruit or 300 mL sports drink
1 cup of fruit salad with 200 g carton fruit-flavored yogurt or custard
200 g carton fruit-flavored yogurt or 300 mL flavored milk and 30–35 g cereal bar
2 crumpets or English muffins with thick spread of peanut butter
250 g tin baked beans on 2 slices of toast
250 g (large) baked potato with cottage cheese or grated cheese filling
150 g thick-crust pizza

Portable carbohydrate-rich foods suitable for the traveling rower
Breakfast cereal (and skim milk powder)
Cereal bars, granola bars
Dried fruit, trail mixes
Rice crackers, dry biscuits plus spreads — jam, honey, etc.
Quick cook noodles and rice
Baked beans
Sports bars
Liquid meal supplements — powder and ready-to-drink tetra packs Sports drink

---

appropriately trained to minimize their measurement error and to understand the limitations of their assessments. These techniques can be used to identify the range of values for body fat and body weight for groups of heavyweight and lightweight rowers, and to monitor the health and performance of individual rowers within this range. Longitudinal profiling of a rower can monitor the development of physical characteristics that are associated with good performance for that individual, as well as identify the changes in physique that can be expected over a season or period of specialized training. For the lightweight rower in particular, physique assessments may allow the estimation of the minimum body fat levels and body weight that can be safely achieved, or to monitor whether the changes in body fat and muscle mass associated with weight loss are appropriate. Of course, it is rec-

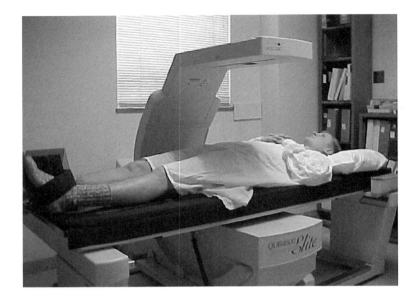

Fig. 9.1 Dual-energy X-ray absorptiometry (DEXA) scan.

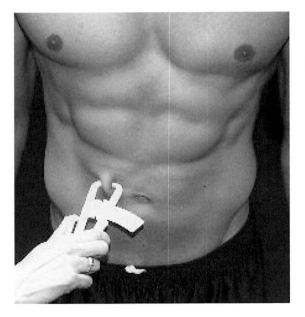

Fig. 9.2 Measurement of skinfold (subcutaneous) fat.

ommended that each rower seek a physique that is compatible with good health and mental well-being, good performances and sound eating patterns in the long-term. Furthermore, it is important to note that it can take many years of training and maturation for a rower to achieve their optimal physique.

Loss of body fat should be achieved through a program of eating and exercise that achieves a sustained and moderate energy deficit. Where dietary restrictions are undertaken, they should not interfere with the rower's ability to fuel training sessions, meet requirements for protein and micronutrients, or place undue stress related to the enjoyment of food or social eating occasions. Dietary strategies that may help a rower achieve loss of body fat are summarized in Table 9.3.

Making weight

Lightweight rowing places weight restrictions on individual competitors and the crew average. For males, the average weight of a crew must not exceed 70 kg and no individual rower can weigh more than 72.5 kg. The limits for females are 57 and 59 kg, respectively. The weigh-in takes place 1–2 h prior to the start of competition and a lightweight rower must weigh-in on the morning of each day they compete. Under the regatta style of competition, the rower might need to weigh-in and race 3–4 times to decide the final outcome.

A number of studies have investigated the weight making practices of lightweight rowers. Typically, the most successful lightweight rowers are tall, with a moderate degree of muscularity and low body fat

Table 9.3 Guidelines for weight loss and making weight in rowers.

General ideas for weight loss
• Fat loss should be achieved via a moderate energy deficit (e.g., 2–4 MJ or 500–1000 kcal·day^{-1}). Energy restriction or additional training should not cause energy availability (total intake minus the energy cost of training) to fall < 30 kcal (189 kJ) per kilogram body mass
• Although reduced energy intake may reduce total protein and carbohydrate intake, the rower should consume these nutrients at strategic times (e.g., immediately after key workouts). This may be achieved by altering the timetable of meals relative to training
• The rower should consume a wide variety of nutrient-dense foods, to meet protein and micronutrient requirements from a reduced energy intake. Micronutrient supplementation should be considered where restricted energy intake is a long-term issue
• A large food volume can be achieved with high-fiber, low energy density foods such as fruits and vegetables. Carbohydrate-rich foods with a low glycemic index, and protein–carbohydrate food matches also help to promote satiety of meals and snacks
• Energy-rich fluids and energy-dense foods should not be consumed in excessive amounts
• A food diary may help to identify the rower's *actual* intake rather than perceived intake, and note the occasions or situations in which the athlete is unable to adhere to their plan
• Rowers should seek professional advice from a sports dietitian, especially where nutritional goals are complex, or where previous dieting behaviors have already caused food-related stress. This may be particularly important for the lightweight rower

Ideas for making weight in lightweight rowers
• The lightweight rower should seek advice from a sports nutrition expert who understands the requirements of lightweight rowing, and the culture and practices of successful rowers. The rower should provide a complete history of their previous practices, with subjective and objective information about the outcomes of these activities
• The basis of a program should be a long-term weight management plan which includes a sensible decision about the weight class that the rower is able to compete in, with safety, health and good performances
• The rower should work with the expert to develop weight and body fat targets that are safe, realistic and effective. These might encompass goals for off-season, heavy training, competition preparation, competition period, weigh-in and actual competition
• Weight loss should be achieved through long-term moderate energy restriction and appropriate exercise, and should be achieved well in advance of the competition period
• A further loss of up to 2–3% body mass might be achieved in the day(s) leading up to competition. A switch to a low-residue diet in comparison to the usual high-fiber diet can be associated with a loss of 0.5–1.0 kg while still allowing the rower to meet fuel needs for competition. Mild dehydration might be used to achieve the final weight target
• The rower should use the time between weigh-in and racing to complete hydration and fuelling goals, especially if intake of fluid and carbohydrate has been less than optimal in the days leading up to the weigh-in

levels. In fact, they are not true "lightweights" at all because their natural or preseason weight is at least 2–4 kg above their designated weight target despite reasonably low body fat levels. Lightweight rowers typically reduce their body mass over the early part of the season to within a kilogram or two of their designated weight requirement by increasing training in conjunction with a reduced intake of fat and energy. The final loss is undertaken over the day(s) before a race, achieved by low residue eating (to reduce gut contents) and by dehydration. These rowers may only be "at weight" at the time of weigh-in, because rehydration strategies after the weigh-in typically cause a weight gain of 1–2 kg before the start of a race. Some lightweight rowers undertake this "weight making" cycle several times over the season, while there are notable cases where rowers practice this strategy only for major competitions such as Olympic Games and World Championships.

Studies of weight making in lightweight rowing show both concerning and reassuring results. At one level there are reports of pathogenic weight loss practices, including fasting and prolonged or recurrent periods of severe restriction of food intake. Strategies to induce dehydration, including fluid restriction combined with saunas or exercise in warm conditions or clothing, are overlaid on these practices. The immediate outcome of adding severe short-term weight loss techniques to an already poor eating pattern ranges from a loss of performance to, in the most extreme cases, death. One fatality among high-level lightweight rowers, just as deaths among other weight making sports such as wrestling, has been reported. The long-term health consequences include an increased risk of disordered eating, loss of lean body mass, interference with bone health and poor nutritional status overall. On the other hand, there is evidence that there are minimal effects on performance when acute weight loss for a race requires only a minor "tweaking" of 1–2 kg against a background of sound eating and training, and the rower practices aggressive refuelling and rehydration in the period between the weigh-in and the race. It is often confronting for sports medicine and science professionals to work with lightweight rowers. Some suggestions are provided in Table 9.3.

Nutrition guidelines for training

Meeting energy requirements

Energy expenditure is increased by high levels of lean body mass, growth (including the response to a resistance training program) and a high-volume training program. These three factors coexist to create very large energy demands — for example, the male rower who faces an increase in training commitment during periods of adolescent growth spurts. Some, but not all rowers with high energy requirements are able to find strategies to meet such demands, and in the case of high training volumes, an adequate carbohydrate supply to fuel the workouts. This achievement is important to allow growth and to maximize the adaptations to training, including the success of specific weight training programs. However, other rowers struggle to meet their requirements. Factors that are implicated in the failure to achieve high energy needs include the following:
• A busy timetable or constant travel which limits access to food
• Inadequate time and opportunity to prepare or even to consume food
• Inability to eat before or during exercise because of the fear of gastrointestinal discomfort
• Depressed appetite following high-intensity training sessions, or because of the general fatigue accompanying a heavy exercise program
• The bulkiness and volume of carbohydrate-rich foods — particularly high-fiber choices
• Inadequate finances to purchase sufficient food or the specialized sports foods that can make high energy intakes more practical

Solutions for addressing these challenges are found in Table 9.4.

Meeting protein and micronutrient requirements

In general, a varied intake of foods within a moderate to high energy allowance provides opportunities for an athlete to meet their needs for macronutrients and micronutrients. Rowers who consume diets that are limited in quantity, variety

Table 9.4 Strategies to assist a rower to achieve a high energy intake.

• The rower should aim for a pattern of small frequent meals each day to achieve an adequate energy intake and promote recovery/adaptation to resistance training and other key training sessions
• A snack providing carbohydrate and protein will enhance recovery after key training sessions as well as contribute to total daily energy intake. Such a snack should also be consumed prior to resistance training sessions. Examples of foods combining these nutrients are provided in Table 9.2
• Carbohydrate should be consumed during prolonged workouts to provide additional fuel as well as contribute to total daily energy intake
• A food diary may help to identify the rower's *actual* intake rather than perceived intake, and note the occasions or situations in which the rower is unable to adhere to their plan of frequent meals and snacks
• The rower is often faced with a chaotic and overcommitted lifestyle. Good skills in time management should see the rower using quieter periods to undertake food shopping and meal preparation activities so that food is available during hectic periods
• During travel, the rower should take a supply of portable and non-perishable snacks that will allow them to continue high-energy eating in a new environment (see Table 9.2 for examples)
• Specialized products such as sports drinks, sports gels and sports bars provide a practical form of carbohydrate during exercise, while sports bars and liquid meal supplements provide an accessible form of carbohydrate and protein for post-exercise recovery
• Energy-containing drinks such as liquid meal supplements, flavored milk, fruit smoothies, sports drinks, soft drinks and juices provide a low-bulk way to consume energy and other important nutrients while meeting fluid needs
• Although fiber intake is important in a healthy diet, excessive intake of high-fiber foods may limit total energy intake or lead to gastrointestinal discomfort. It may be necessary to moderate intake of wholegrain or fiber-enriched versions of foods

or both, are at risk of failing to consume key nutrients at strategic times (e.g., recovery eating), or of consuming suboptimal intakes of protein and micronutrients. This situation mostly applies to lightweight rowers who struggle with their weight making goals. Although protein needs may be increased by heavy training, protein does not appear to be an "at risk" nutrient, unless dietary variety and energy intake are severely restricted. The micronutrient most likely to be at risk of suboptimal intake is iron. Iron requirements are increased not only by growth and the onset of menstruation in females, but may also need to take into account a small increase in iron loss related to training. Although iron losses from exercise-related hemolysis are generally associated with contact and foot-strike sports, a rower may incur an increase in gut iron losses because of the effects of anti-inflammatory drugs or gastrointestinal problems causing malabsorption. Iron lost in sweat may also be a cause of increased iron losses. In general, however, most cases of iron deficiency occur because of inadequate intake of iron from bioavailable sources. Iron supplementation may be required to prevent or treat iron deficiency in rowers, but should only be taken as part of a supervised program that also involves dietary changes to enhance iron intake.

Hydration before, during and after training sessions

Although competitive events in rowing involve sustained high-intensity workloads, the brief duration of a single race is unlikely to be associated with levels of fluid loss or fuel depletion that are limiting for performance. The exceptions to this principle are lightweight rowers who dehydrate and restrict their food intake in order to make weight, and rowers who are involved in a series of races over a short time period with inadequate time or opportunity for recovery between. By contrast, training sessions are undertaken at moderate and high intensities over prolonged periods—factors that cause high sweat losses and high rates of glycogen utilization. As a result, strategies to replace fluid and carbohydrate during training are potentially important, but may not be appreciated by rowers who perceive that they participate in a non-endurance sport.

All the on-water sessions undertaken by two groups of well-trained rowers over a week of training in different climates were monitored. In hot conditions, workouts resulted in mean sweat rates of ~2 L·h^{-1} for males and 1400 mL·h^{-1} for females. The same training undertaken by a matched group of rowers in cool conditions caused mean hourly sweat losses of 1200 and 800 mL·h^{-1}, respectively. Although the rowers were aware of the need to consume fluid during training, their intake was limited by the need to carry their own supplies out on the boat, and by the need to stop rowing in order to drink. A number of rowers incurred fluid deficits of at least 2–3% of body mass per session, even under cool conditions. Practical issues in improving fluid intake include organizing sufficient "drink breaks" between pieces in the session, and having adequate supplies on the boat or with the coach. Of course, gastrointestinal discomfort may limit total fluid intake during rowing workouts involving high-intensity pieces.

There are few studies of the effects of fluid intake on rowing performance in training or competition. Dehydration has been examined mostly in the case of "weight making" practices of lightweights but these results need to be interpreted in light of the restricted food intake that typically accompanies dehydration techniques. Nevertheless, it makes sense for the rower to try to minimize the fluid deficit that accrues during a training session—typically, a goal of < 2% body mass is recommended. Following each workout, the rower should replace the remaining fluid deficit in preparation for future sessions. When sweat losses are high, an intake equivalent to ~125–150% of the volume of the fluid deficit over the next 2–4 h is typically required to restore fluid balance in the face of continuing urine losses. In addition, sodium replacement should occur through the intake of electrolyte containing drinks (e.g., sports drinks, oral rehydration solutions) or salt added to meals and snacks. This rehydration strategy may also be used by lightweight rowers in the period after their weigh-in.

Fuelling before, during and after training sessions

High-intensity rowing training is characterized by high rates of carbohydrate oxidation and,

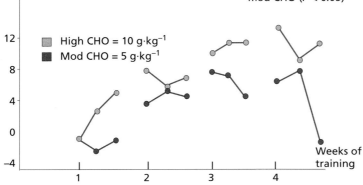

Average power (W)
% Change from day 1

Power over 4 weeks: significantly greater with
high vs. mod CHO
Day 26: Power 7.8% higher in high vs. mod CHO
($P < 0.05$)
Change from day 1 to 26: 10.7% high vs. 1.6%
mod CHO ($P < 0.05$)

High CHO = 10 g·kg^{-1}
Mod CHO = 5 g·kg^{-1}

Weeks of
training

Fig. 9.3 Changes in mean power output during rowing ergometer training session ($3 \times 2500\,\text{m}$) undertake 3 times a week when collegiate rowers undertook 4 weeks of training on energy matched diets providing moderate ($5\,\text{g·kg}^{-1}\text{·day}^{-1}$) or high ($10\,\text{g·kg}^{-1}\text{·day}^{-1}$) intakes of carbohydrate (CHO). From Simonsen *et al.* (1991) with permission.

presumably, substantial depletion of muscle glycogen stores. Therefore, strategies that increase carbohydrate availability during workouts might be expected to enhance training performance. These strategies include a high carbohydrate eating pattern in general, as well as specific intake of carbohydrate before, during and in the recovery from key training sessions. Benefits might include better maintenance of muscle workloads as well as reduced levels of neuromuscular fatigue — an interaction that is important to a sport that involves coordinated technique and motor control such as rowing. Specific studies need to be undertaken to confirm these benefits. As pointed out in the case of fluid intake, there are some practical impediments to consuming carbohydrate during a heavy training session. However, the use of sports drinks, sports gels and bars can assist the rower to refuel during a workout. Table 9.2 provides suggestions that would allow a rower to consume an intake of ~50 g carbohydrate per hour of training.

Even if better performance of a single session of rowing can be demonstrated through better fuel availability, it takes particular patience and large resources to investigate whether the repetition of these strategies translates into better long-term training adaptations and competition performance. In one such study, two groups of collegiate rowers completed a 4 week training program on energy-matched diets providing either 5 or 10 g·kg^{-1} body mass of carbohydrate per day. Monitoring of muscle glycogen content showed that the moderate carbohydrate group maintained muscle carbohydrate stores, while the high carbohydrate diet promoted an increase in stores over the duration of the study. At the evening workout on days 1, 3 and 5 of each week, the rowers undertook $3 \times 2500\,\text{m}$ time trials on a rowing ergometer. In the moderate carbohydrate group, power during the time trials was maintained over the 4 W, leading to an overall improvement of 1.6% at the end of the training block. Meanwhile, the high carbohydrate group showed an improvement of 10.7% over the same time frame (Fig. 9.3). This study shows that a higher carbohydrate intake supports superior training adaptations and performance in heavily training athletes, but suggests that a reasonable time frame is needed before the differences become detectable.

Apart from direct enhancement of training performance, there may be other advantages to providing nutritional support during a workout. Prolonged and high-intensity exercise is associated with disturbances to the immune system, particularly during the post-exercise period. Some studies have reported that these disturbances are reduced when carbohydrate is consumed during prolonged exercise than when carbohydrate levels are low. However, the ideal study that shows that chronic carbohydrate support during training leads to a reduced frequency or severity of illness in rowers is yet to be undertaken. Notwithstanding these limitations, the current literature suggests that good health and protection of the immune system may be a secondary but substantial benefit of carbohydrate intake during heavy periods of training.

Finally, although total carbohydrate intake appears to be the most important dietary factor in promoting refuelling over the day, the timing of intake of carbohydrate may be important for rowers who undertake several sessions of training in a day. Effective rates of muscle glycogen resynthesis do not occur after exercise until there has been an intake of substantial amounts of carbohydrate (e.g., at least $1\,g\cdot kg^{-1}$ body mass). When there is less than 8 h between training sessions, it makes sense to maximize refuelling between workouts by commencing carbohydrate intake as practical during recovery. If it is not convenient to eat a meal immediately after training, carbohydrate-rich snacks or drinks providing at least $1\,g\cdot kg^{-1}$ should be consumed (and repeated every hour) until the normal meal routine is resumed. Often, poor appetite, a busy lifestyle or poor access to appropriate foods interfere with this routine. Other issues of recovery can be built into post-training snacks and meals by choosing combinations of carbohydrate-rich foods and drinks that also provide protein, fluids and electrolytes (Table 9.2).

Nutrition guidelines for competition

High-level competitions in rowing are generally held as multiday regattas, with the duration ranging from three-day World Cup events to the week-long program of the Olympics and World Championships. Events are completed as a series of heats or preliminaries, repechages for additional qualification, semi-finals and finals. At high-level competition, a crew may need to race 3–4 times over 4–7 days before final outcomes are decided. At lower levels of

competition, rowers may compete over a single day of racing.

Fuelling for competition

Adequate carbohydrate and fluid levels are important for optimal performance, but are not likely to be limiting for a single event if adequate pre-race preparation and post-race recovery from previous races has taken place. This calls for a planned approach to eating for a race, especially when the rower is competing in events away from their home base. A key part of the competition eating plan is to understand the rower's real energy and fuel needs over the racing period. The competition program will involve warm-ups and cool-down activities in addition to the actual race program, as well as continued training on rest days. However, the energy cost of racing activities is usually substantially less than the usual training program. Therefore, strategic refuelling and rehydration practices may need to be organized within an eating program that achieves an adjusted energy intake. This may be particularly important for the lightweight rower who must stay below a weight target.

For some rowers, racing is often a time of unnecessary gain of body fat, as the athlete "overfuels" themselves in the belief that this will assist their race performance. Overeating can also occur during racing periods because the young athlete is away from their normal supervised nutrition plan, or because the rower is eating in response to the nervousness and anxiety generated by competition. By contrast, other rowers with a busy race schedule and extensive travel commitments find their access to food is limited. Poor food availability at the event location and the distraction of racing activities can all interfere with the achievement of a well-chosen eating routine. In such cases the rower will unnecessarily lose weight over the competition period, as well as fail to achieve optimal recovery strategies between races.

The rower can prepare adequate muscle glycogen stores for racing by ensuring at least 24–36 h tapered training and high carbohydrate intake (7–$10\,g\cdot kg^{-1}$ body mass per day) in the lead up to a race. This equates to a daily intake of 400–650 g carbohydrate for a typical 65–70 kg female rower and 600–900 g for a 90 kg male rower. Such targets will also ensure optimal refuelling between races in a multiday program. Lightweight rowers may need to moderate their total intake of food in the day(s) leading up to a race, and consume low-residue forms of carbohydrate-rich foods to find a compromise between achieving fuel needs and meeting their weight target.

Pre-race and post-race eating

The daily racing routine should start with a high carbohydrate pre-race meal, which the rower should choose from a range of familiar foods and following a plan that has been fine-tuned from previous racing experience (Table 9.2). The goals of the pre-race meal are to top up body glycogen stores, particularly liver stores which may be depleted by an overnight fast. Fluids consumed with this meal and over the hours prior to a race allow the rower to ensure that they are well-hydrated for events undertaken in hot weather. Above all, the rower should choose a menu that ensures that they feel comfortable and at low risk of suffering gastrointestinal problems. Typically, heavyweight rowers consume a pre-race breakfast 1–3 h before commencing pre-race warm-ups. However, lightweight rowers can usually only consume significant amounts of fluid and food following their weigh-in. During and after warm-ups, and in recovery between races on the same program, carbohydrate-containing drinks (e.g., sports drinks) and light carbohydrate foods (sports bars, fruit, gels) may be consumed to maintain body carbohydrate supplies and prevent hunger.

After the competition session is completed, the rower should consume a nutrient-rich snack or meal to meet recovery goals of refuelling, repairing muscle damage and rehydration. As outlined in the section above, post-exercise recovery may be enhanced by speedy intake of foods and/or drinks providing a source of carbohydrate, protein, fluids and electrolytes. Many rowers take a selection of portable snacks and drinks to the competition venue to allow refuelling and rehydration after each event and during the competition program. Issues such as storage facilities, appetite appeal during a heavy racing program, and the need to comply with drug testing protocols (i.e., only accepting food and drinks from sealed containers) often determine the suitable choices. Typical choices include specialized sports foods (sports drinks, liquid meal supplements, bars and gels) as well as cereal and granola bars, fresh and dried fruit, jelly confectionery and sandwiches. When regattas are held in hot locations, rowers should have ready access to a supply of fluids over the day, and should monitor hydration levels to combat sweat losses from the environment as well as the specific losses during events and warm-ups.

Supplements and sports foods for rowing

The sports world is filled with pills, potions and powders that claim to enhance performance, improve recovery, increase muscle mass and reduce body fat levels. Although only a small proportion of these claims have credible scientific support, surveys show that most athletes are enthusiastic consumers of such products. Some supplements and sports foods offer real advantages to the athlete.

Table 9.5 summarizes the products that have scientific evidence of potential benefits in the training and competition programs of rowers. Unfortunately, in many cases, the evidence is of benefits to the type of issues faced by rowers rather than specific studies of the training and competition outcomes of real rowers. Therefore, there is a need for further specific studies to confirm the theories summarized in the table. Of course, it is the appropriate use of the product as much as the product itself that leads to the beneficial outcome. Therefore, rowers need to be well educated about specific situations and strategies for the use of supplements and sports foods, rather than considering them to be "magic solutions" per se. Furthermore, any decision to use sports supplements or foods should consider the evidence for real or even placebo-driven benefits versus the risk of side effects. A real concern for rowers who compete under anti-doping codes, is that the products may contain substances as contaminants or undeclared ingredients that will cause a positive doping outcome. Supplement use, even when it provides a true performance advantage, is an expense that the rower must acknowledge and

Table 9.5 Sports foods and supplements that are of likely benefit to rowers.

Product	Comment
Used to achieve nutrition goals	
Sports drinks	To refuel and rehydrate during prolonged workouts, and for post-training rehydration
Sports gels	Convenient and compact carbohydrate source that can be carried for use during prolonged rowing sessions or dry-land training
Sports bars	Convenient, portable and easy to consume source of carbohydrate, protein and micronutrients for a pre-race meal, high-energy diet or post-exercise recovery Convenient and compact source of energy and nutrients during travel
Liquid meal supplements	As for sports bars Low residue food that can be used as a pre-event food by lightweight rowers
Vitamin/mineral supplements	Supplemental source of micronutrients for travel when food supply is unreliable Supplemental source of micronutrients during prolonged periods of energy restriction
Strong potential for ergogenic benefit	
Caffeine	May enhance performance of rowing events when consumed pre-race, but further sports-specific studies are needed to investigate the timing and range of doses that are effective. There is some evidence that small to moderate doses of caffeine ($1–3\,mg\cdot kg^{-1}$) are as effective as larger doses ($5–6\,mg\cdot kg^{-1}$). This may reduce the risk of side effects such as tremor and/or anxiety affecting technique or problems with post-race sleep
Bicarbonate or citrate	Acute use of bicarbonate or citrate to increase blood buffering capacity (e.g., $300\,mg\cdot k^{-1}g^{-1}$ BM bicarbonate loading or $500\,mg\cdot kg^{-1}$ BM citrate 1–2 h pre-race) may enhance the performance of rowing events because of an increased tolerance to production of H^+ ions via anaerobic glycolysis. Further field studies are needed with high-level athletes to confirm benefits. Risk of gastrointestinal problems should be noted. Rowers who intend to load for a series of events over a day or consecutive days (e.g., heats and finals) should consider a chronic loading protocol (e.g., $500\,mg\cdot kg^{-1}\cdot day^{-1}$ for 5 days spread into a series of doses over the day) to achieve a more sustained increase in blood buffering capacity
Creatine	Creatine supplementation enhances the performance of exercise involving repeated high-intensity work bouts with short recovery intervals. Creatine loading ($4 \times 5\,g$ doses for 5 days) and maintenance ($2–5\,g\cdot day^{-1}$) may enhance adaptations to interval and resistance training. Acute weight gain of ~1 kg makes it unsuitable for most lightweight rowers

BM, body mass.

prioritize appropriately within their total budget. At best, sports foods and supplements may provide a small but valuable part of the rower's overall nutrition, but they cannot replace the benefits of well-chosen eating plans.

References and recommended reading

Bruce, C.R., Anderson, M.E., Fraser, S.F., *et al.* (2000) Enhancement of 2000-m rowing performance after caffeine ingestion. *Medicine and Science in Sports and Exercise* **32**, 1958–1963.

Burke, L.M. (2007a) Rowing and swimming. *Practical Sports Nutrition*, pp. 141–168. Human Kinetics, Champaign, IL.

Burke, L.M. (2007b) Weight making sports. *Practical Sports Nutrition*, pp. 289–313. Human Kinetics, Champaign, IL.

Chwalbinska-Moneta, J. (2003) Effect of creatine supplementation on aerobic performance and anaerobic capacity in elite rowers in the course of endurance training. *International Journal of Sport Nutrition and Exercise Metabolism* **13**, 173–183.

Maughan, R.J., Burke, L.M & Coyle, E.F. (2004) *Foods, Nutrition and Sports Performance II*. Routledge, London.

McNaughton, L.R. & Cedaro, R. (1991) The effect of sodium bicarbonate on rowing ergometer performance in elite rowers. *Australian Journal of Science and Medicine in Sport* **23**, 66–69.

Simonsen, J.C., Sherman, W.M., Lamb, D.R., Dernbach, A.R., Doyle, J.A. & Strauss, R. (1991) Dietary carbohydrate, muscle glycogen, and power output during rowing training. *Journal of Applied Physiology* **70**, 1500–1505.

Slater, G.J., Rice, A.J., Tanner, R., Sharpe, K., Jenkins, D. & Hahn, A.G. (2006a) Impact of two different body management strategies on repeat rowing performance. *Medicine and Science in Sports and Exercise* **38**, 138–146.

Slater, G.J., Rice, A.J., Tanner, R., Sharpe, K., Jenkins, D. & Hahn, A.G (2006b) Acute weight loss followed by an aggressive nutritional recovery strategy has little impact on on-water rowing performance. *British Journal of Sports Medicine* **40**, 55–59.

Talbott, S.M. & Shapses, S.A. (1998) Fasting and energy intake influence bone turnover in lightweight male rowers. *International Journal of Sport Nutrition* **8**, 377–387.

Chapter 10
The senior oarsman

C. Yoshiga

Health

Rowing was one of the first, if not the first, organized sport and involves participants ranging from early adolescence to advanced age. Consequently, rowing offered an early opportunity for evaluating longevity associated with vigorous physical exercise. Several studies show that rowing continued throughout life attenuates the age-related deterioration of physiologic functions and that it may favor life expectancy. In 1928 Pierre de Coubertin published a brochure entitled *La cure d'aviron* (health through rowing), and at 72 was still an active oarsman.

Correspondence to *The Times* on October 10, 1869 claimed that the University Regatta was a national folly as rowers were exposed to permanent danger to their health that could even threaten their lifespan. A study that evaluated these dark prophecies, however, showed that oarsmen participating in the Oxford–Cambridge regatta lived about 2 years longer than the British life expectancy at that time. Harvard University oarsmen have also been reported to live 3–6 years longer than the US life expectancy in the early 19th century. The only contradictory finding of a somewhat lower average age at death of Cambridge University crew oarsmen than in a random group of people (67.1 vs. 67.4 years) from the same time period can be attributed to their engagement in World War I. Nevertheless, having considered the interference of world affairs, the death rate from cardiovascular disease is lower in oarsmen than in a random control group of people

and such observations are now available from participants in a large range of activities. Thus, in perspective studies there is a direct relationship between lifespan and physical activity including a reduced prevalence of certain types of cancer, such as colon cancer. An early observation by Morris was that the conductors of London's double decker buses live longer than the drivers and similar observations made in Finland show a progressive increase in the lifespan of international championship participants, depending on the type of sport, ranging from power sports to ball games and endurance events. However, it may be that such comparisons reflect evaluations of participants with different genetic make-up. In that light, a specific polymorphism in the gene encoding the angiontensin-converting enzyme resulting in low range values of angiotensin in plasma is overrepresented in successful competitive Australian rowers. Also, this "insertion" allele is associated with elite endurance performance among high-altitude mountaineers. On the other hand, the "deletion" allele producing relatively high levels of angiotensin has been identified as a risk factor for the development of cardiovascular diseases. Thus, the findings of better life expectancy in rowers may reflect a genetic selection of these individuals in addition to the beneficial effect of chronic participation in rowing per se.

Height

With aging, body height decreases by approximately 2 cm because of the progressive curvature of the

Table 10.1 Indicative body dimensions and cardiorespiratory variables among older and young oarsmen and sedentary men matched for height and weight ($n = 17$). $\dot{V}O_{2max}$, maximal oxygen uptake; $\dot{V}O_2$, oxygen uptake; [La⁻], blood lactate concentration; HR_{max}, maximal heart rate; HR, heart rate; $\dot{V}_{Emax}$, maximal ventilation.

	Older oarsmen	Older sedentary men	Young oarsmen	Young sedentary men
Age (years)	64 ± 4	65 ± 3	22 ± 2	23 ± 2
Body fat (%)	18 ± 4	23 ± 4	12 ± 4	17 ± 4
Fat free mass (kg)	56 ± 5	53 ± 5	61 ± 4	57 ± 5
$\dot{V}O_{2max}$ (L·min⁻¹)	3.0 ± 0.4	2.2 ± 0.3	4.2 ± 0.3	3.1 ± 0.5
$\dot{V}O_2$ at [La⁻] of 4 mmol·L⁻¹ (L·min⁻¹)	2.6 ± 0.3	1.8 ± 0.3	3.7 ± 0.4	2.7 ± 0.5
HR_{max} (beats·min⁻¹)	176 ± 13	166 ± 9	198 ± 8	201 ± 9
HR at [La⁻] of 4 mmol·L⁻¹ (beats·min⁻¹)	163 ± 12	157 ± 11	177 ± 12	177 ± 11
Maximal oxygen pulse (mL·beat⁻¹)	17.2 ± 2.3	13.5 ± 2.0	21.6 ± 1.8	15.4 ± 2.5
Oxygen pulse at [La⁻] of 4 mmol·L⁻¹ (mL·beat⁻¹)	17.0 ± 0.9	11.5 ± 0.9	20.7 ± 1.0	15.0 ± 1.1
$\dot{V}_{Emax}$ (L·min⁻¹)	117 ± 17	74 ± 13	162 ± 18	84 ± 17
[La⁻] after maximal exercise (mmol·L⁻¹)	8.3 ± 1.0	7.9 ± 1.1	10.9 ± 1.1	10.0 ± 1.2
Rowing performance 2000 m (s)	489 ± 16		451 ± 12	

spine and osteoporotic collapse of the vertebrae. This decrease in body height develops from the age of ~40 to ~60 years even in people who continue to be active, and so there is no reported difference in height between older oarsmen and sedentary men. Likely reflecting the increasing height of the population, older oarsmen are shorter than their young counterparts but there is a lack of longitudinal studies evaluating the effect of regular rowing on osteoporosis and the aging-related decline of the length of the spinal column.

Osteoporosis

Peak bone mass is established in both men and women around the age of 30 years and subsequently declines by ~0.5% per year in men and by ~1% per year in women. The decline in bone mass observed throughout life contributes to the elevated incidence of osteoporotic fractures. Physical activity, especially weight-bearing activity, is an essential requirement for maintained bone mass.

Body mass

As body mass increases with age, probably because of reduced physical activity, the risks of falling,

fracture and limb disability, as well as morbidity from major chronic diseases and even mortality, are increased. Regular rowing provides sufficient volume and intensity of physical activity for the maintenance of low body mass in elderly people. There is greater prevalence of obesity with age, which is linked with numerous chronic diseases including type II diabetes, hypertension and cardiac disease, and thereby to mortality. Even though body fat is higher in older compared with that in young oarsmen (18% vs. 12%; Table 10.1), it is similar to that of young sedentary men and lower than in sedentary men matched for age and body size (18% vs. 23%; Table 10.2).

Aging is also characterized by a decrease in fat free mass. In spite of lower fat free mass, older oarsmen have a larger fat free mass than elderly sedentary men or habitual runners, and maintain a fat free mass similar to young sedentary men. Thus, rowing contributes to attenuate the age-related loss of fat free mass and reduces obesity and therefore morbidity associated with chronic diseases.

Aerobic capacity

Elderly individuals who engage in regular physical activity have a slower decline in $\dot{V}O_{2max}$ compared

Table 10.2 Body dimensions and cardiorespiratory variables among older, young performance-matched, and qualified oarsmen. $\dot{V}O_{2max}$, maximal oxygen uptake; $\dot{V}O_2$, oxygen uptake; [La⁻], blood lactate concentration; HR_{max}, maximal heart rate; HR, heart rate; $\dot{V}_{Emax}$, maximal ventilation.

	Older oarsmen	Young performance-matched oarsmen	Young qualified oarsmen
Age (years)	62 ± 2	21 ± 1	22 ± 1
Body height (cm)	174 ± 4	172 ± 4	181 ± 4
Body mass (kg)	72 ± 5	71 ± 6	80 ± 8
Body fat (%)	17 ± 3	17 ± 4	11 ± 2
Fat free mass (kg)	60 ± 5	59 ± 4	71 ± 5
$\dot{V}O_{2max}$ (L·min⁻¹)	3.3 ± 0.4	3.1 ± 0.3	5.1 ± 0.4
$\dot{V}O_2$ at [La⁻] of 4 mmol·L⁻¹ (L·min⁻¹)	2.5 ± 0.4	2.5 ± 0.4	4.4 ± 0.4
HR_{max} (beats·min⁻¹)	176 ± 5	188 ± 7	189 ± 7
HR at [La⁻] of 4 mmol·L⁻¹ (beats·min⁻¹)	149 ± 11	165 ± 12	175 ± 8
Maximal oxygen pulse (mL·beat⁻¹)	19.5 ± 2.1	17.6 ± 1.8	26.9 ± 2.2
Oxygen pulse at [La⁻] of 4 mmol·L⁻¹ (mL·beat⁻¹)	16.8 ± 0.9	15.6 ± 1.1	25.1 ± 1.0
$\dot{V}_{Emax}$ (L·min⁻¹)	121 ± 15	126 ± 13	178 ± 10
[La⁻] after maximal exercise (mmol·L⁻¹)	8.4 ± 1.0	9.8 ± 1.6	10.3 ± 1.8
Rowing performance 2000 m (s)	495 ± 14	494 ± 13	387 ± 7

with sedentary elderly people. Elderly oarsmen have a lower $\dot{V}O_{2max}$ compared with young oarsmen (3.0 vs. 4.1 L·min⁻¹; Table 10.1) but their $\dot{V}O_{2max}$ is larger than in sedentary men matched for age and body size (3.0 vs. 2.2 L·min⁻¹; Fig. 10.1) and similar to young sedentary men. Thus, regular rowing continued in advanced age slows the aging-related decline in aerobic fitness.

The decay of cardiorespiratory function with age is also represented by a greater increase in blood lactate at a given submaximal exercise intensity. Older oarsmen, however, achieve a given lactate level at a higher exercise intensity, expressed by $\dot{V}O_2$, compared with sedentary men matched for age and body size (blood lactate of 4 mmol·L⁻¹ at 2.6 vs. 1.8 L·min⁻¹). Also, elderly competitive oarsmen possess a $\dot{V}O_2$ similar to young oarsmen matched for 2000 m rowing performance time (Table 10.2).

In addition, $\dot{V}_{Emax}$ decreases with age, which might be explained by loss of elasticity of the lung tissue and the chest wall, both of which demand more work associated with breathing. While neither rowing nor regular running prevent the age-associated decrease in $\dot{V}_{Emax}$ (117 vs. 162 L·min⁻¹ in

elderly oarsmen compared with young oarsmen), rowing performed on a daily basis is associated with an attenuated age-related decrease in respiratory function when matched for age and body size (117 vs. 74 L·min⁻¹; Table 10.1). Interestingly, elderly oarsmen exhibit a $\dot{V}_{Emax}$ similar to young oarsmen matched for rowing performance and body size (121 vs. 124 L·min⁻¹; Table 10.2).

Heart rate

Heart rate (HR) is a simple but informative parameter both in clinical and physiologic exercise settings. As HR increases nearly linearly with work rate to maximal exercise, this relationship is used widely to predict work capacity, or $\dot{V}O_{2max}$, from values derived at a submaximal work intensity. HR_{max} decreases progressively with aging and is lower in older compared with young oarsmen and sedentary men (176 vs. 201 and 198 beats·min⁻¹, respectively; Table 10.1, Fig. 10.1). However, regular rowing has a role in blunting the age-associated decline of HR_{max}, as demonstrated by higher HR_{max} in older oarsmen than older sedentary men (166 beats·min⁻¹).

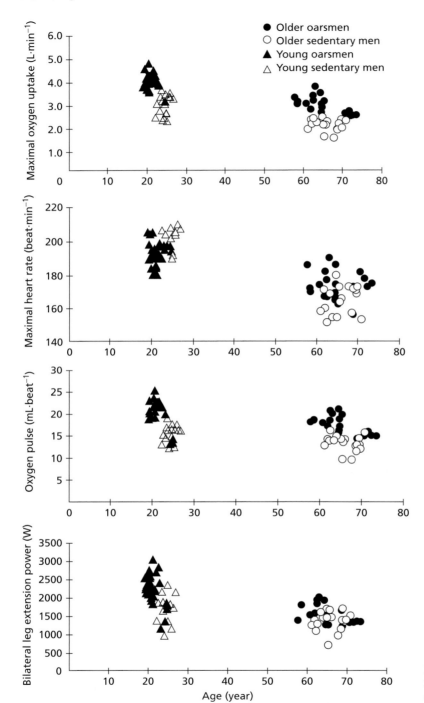

Fig. 10.1 Oxygen uptake, heart rate, oxygen pulse and bilateral leg extension power related to age.

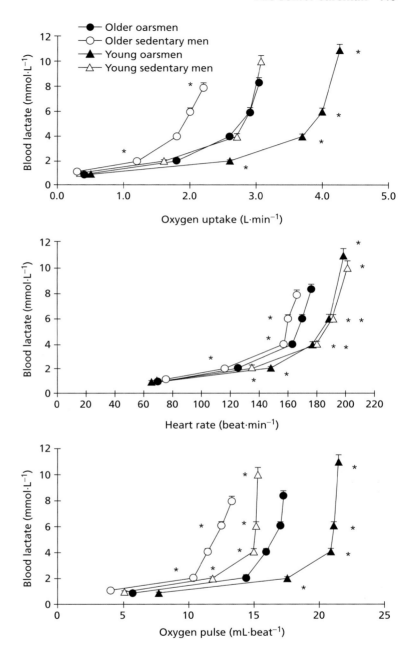

Fig. 10.2 Oxygen uptake, heart rate and oxygen pulse response to incremental exercise. The difference from older oarsmen is indicated by *.

Similarly, with the reduction in $\dot{V}O_{2max}$, HR at a submaximal workrate increases with age, as indicated by the achievement of a given blood lactate level at a lower HR in older oarsmen compared with young oarsmen with similar rowing performance (149 vs. 165 beats·min^{-1} at 4 mmol·L^{-1}). On the other hand, an age-associated decrease in HR at submaximal work intensity is modified by habitual rowing training, as demonstrated by the achievement of a blood lactate of 4 mmol·L^{-1} at a higher HR in older oarsmen compared with older sedentary men (163 vs. 157 beats·min^{-1}; Fig. 10.2).

The seated position elicits a lower HR response during rowing compared with running at comparable exercise intensity both in older and young men and women. This rowing-induced reduction in the HR response to exercise is associated with an expanded central blood volume as shown by a higher plasma atrial natriuretic peptide (ANP; 131 vs. 100 pg·mL^{-1}, released by atrial stretch) and central venous pressure (CVP; 3.3 vs. −5.2 mmHg) compared with running. Consequently, when HR$_{max}$ predicted by the traditional equation that 220 minus age is applied for estimating exercise intensity relative to $\dot{V}O_{2max}$, the flat relationship between HR and $\dot{V}O_2$ during rowing should be taken into consideration in order not to prescribe a too large workload.

Structure and function of the heart

The weight of the heart increases by an average 1 g·year^{-1} in men and 1.5 g·year^{-1} in women, reflecting some degree of left ventricular hypertrophy, even in subjects apparently free of hypertension. Regular rowing induces favorable alterations of the heart, as shown by a cardiac hypertrophy in older oarsmen compared with sedentary men (septum thickness, 11 vs. 9 mm; posterior wall thickness, 9 vs. 8 mm; left ventricular mass, 227 vs. 205 g; left ventricular mass index, 127 vs. 103 g·m^{-2}). In addition, rowing continued into advanced age offers protection against deterioration of cardiovascular function with age, as demonstrated by enhanced systolic function (left ventricular shortening fraction, 0.45 vs. 0.36).

With regard to cardiac function and systemic hemodynamics, the maximal cardiac output declines with advancing age because of a decrease in stroke volume. The oxygen pulse ($\dot{V}O_2$/HR) is used as an index of stroke volume. The age-related decline in stroke volume is not completely averted by regular rowing, demonstrated by a lower value in older compared with young oarsmen, but this reduction is attenuated as demonstrated by a higher oxygen pulse in older oarsmen compared with sedentary men matched for age and body size (17 vs. 12 mL·beat^{-1} at a blood lactate level of 4 mmol·L^{-1}; 17 vs. 14 mL·beat^{-1} at maximal effort; Table 10.1, Figs 10.1 & 10.2). Additionally, there is similar oxygen pulse between older and young oarsmen with similar 2000 m rowing performance time.

Blood lactate concentration

Aging reduces muscle oxidative capacity, capillarization and oxidative enzymes activity; changes that are reflected in the reduced blood lactate concentration immediately after maximal exercise in sedentary men and even in vigorously trained endurance runners and cyclists. Similarly, the age-associated reduction in maximal blood lactate is not prevented by lifelong rowing as shown by lower values in older compared with young oarsmen and sedentary men (8.3 vs. 10.9 and 10.0 mmol·L^{-1}; Table 10.1, Fig. 10.2). Nevertheless, the higher maximal blood lactate values in older oarsmen compared with sedentary men matched for age and body size (7.9 mmol·L^{-1}) suggest that rowing carried out throughout life attenuates the age-associated decline in skeletal muscle adaptation to physical training.

Risk factors of coronary artery disease

Dyslipidoproteinemia (i.e., elevated concentrations of total cholesterol [TC], triglycerides [TG], low-density lipoprotein cholesterol [LDL-C] and a reduced concentration of high-density lipoprotein cholesterol [HDL-C] in plasma) are risk factors for coronary artery disease. The LDL-C is implicated in plaque formation in blood vessels, while the HDL-C is involved in plaque removal. Thus, the ratio of LDL-C to HDL-C, or that of TC to HDL-C (i.e., the atherosclerosis index) is applied to evaluate individual risks for coronary artery disease. Also, aging is considered as one of the secondary risk factors for development of coronary artery disease. Lifelong rowing fosters attenuation in risk factors for coronary artery disease in aged men, which is grounded on a lower atherosclerosis index in older oarsmen (LDL-C:HDL-C, 1.7; TC:HDL-C, 3.1) compared with both older and young sedentary men (LDL-C:HDL-C, 2.1 and 2.1; TC:HDL-C, 3.6 and 3.5, respectively).

Aging is associated with a progressive increase in body fat, which results from a declining level of physical activity. Leptin is a protein produced by "the obesity (ob) gene" and its secretion from adipose tissue to the circulation is considered to signal the brain regarding the size and the nutritional status of adipose tissue, a signal that seems to be lost or inhibited in people who become very fat. Rowing continued into advanced age has a protective effect on the age-associated increase in fat mass and serum concentration of leptin, as reflected by the lower leptin values in older oarsmen compared with older sedentary men matched for body size (fat mass, 13 vs. 16 kg; serum leptin, 2.5 vs. 4.1 ng·mL^{-1}, respectively; Table 10.3). Thus, the serum concentration of leptin is correlated to percentage body fat ($r = 0.60$) and cross-sectional area of leg fat.

Insulin is an important hormone that reduces glucose circulating in the blood by facilitating its transport into the cells. There is an inverse relationship between the level of habitual physical activity and the incidence of type II diabetes. Regular rowing benefits the insulin-stimulated whole-body and skeletal muscle glucose uptake as shown by a lower fasting plasma glucose and insulin in older oarsmen compared with older sedentary men (glucose, 5.3 vs. 5.8 mmol·L^{-1}; insulin, 6.9 vs. 8.7 pmol·L^{-1}, respectively; Table 10.3).

Risk factors of diabetes mellitus

Diabetes is a disorder of carbohydrate metabolism characterized by hyperglycemia and the incidence of type II diabetes increases with advancing age.

Skeletal muscle structure and function

As the rate of protein synthesis declines with aging, skeletal muscle size decreases as shown by the reductions in arm, leg and limb mass even in the

Table 10.3 Metabolic variables. TC, total cholesterol; TG, triglyceride; LDL-, low-density lipoprotein cholesterol; HDL-C, high-density lipoprotein cholesterol.

	Older oarsmen	Older sedentary men	Young oarsmen	Young sedentary men
TC (mmol·L^{-1})	5.2 ± 0.2	5.2 ± 0.4	4.1 ± 0.6	4.8 ± 0.6
TG (mmol·L^{-1})	1.4 ± 0.4	1.3 ± 0.4	0.9 ± 0.3	0.9 ± 0.4
LDL-C (mmol·L^{-1})	2.9 ± 0.4	3.0 ± 0.6	2.0 ± 0.7	2.9 ± 0.7
HDL-C (mmol·L^{-1})	1.7 ± 0.2	1.5 ± 0.2	1.4 ± 0.2	1.6 ± 0.3
LDL-C : HDL-C	1.7 ± 0.2	2.1 ± 0.3	1.3 ± 0.4	2.1 ± 0.4
TC : HDL-C	3.1 ± 0.2	3.6 ± 0.3	2.6 ± 0.4	3.5 ± 0.4
Serum leptin (ng·mL^{-1})	2.5 ± 0.8	4.1 ± 0.8		
Plasma glucose (mmol·L^{-1})	95 ± 6	105 ± 5		
Plasma insulin (pmol·L^{-1})	6.9 ± 0.3	8.7 ± 0.4		

Table 10.4 Bilateral leg extension power and the area of leg extensor muscle.

	Bilateral leg extension power (W)	Area of leg extensor muscle (cm²)	Leg extension power per muscle area (W·cm^{-2})
Older oarsmen	1675 ± 200	77.8 ± 5.4	20.9 ± 2.0
Older sedentary men	1261 ± 196	68.4 ± 5.1	19.9 ± 2.1
Young oarsmen	2358 ± 204		
Young sedentary men	1483 ± 173		
Older oarsmen	1693 ± 205		
Young performance-matched oarsmen	1667 ± 212		
Young qualified oarsmen	2533 ± 225		

endurance trained elderly person. Regular rowing has a profound effect in preventing muscle wasting in older men demonstrated by a larger area of leg extensor muscle compared with older sedentary men (78 vs. 68 cm²; Table 10.4). This favorable influence of rowing on muscular morphology may be attributed to an increase of especially the type I fiber area while aging has a detrimental effect on type II muscle fibers.

The skeletal muscle structural changes associated with aging are also reflected in the arm, leg and back strength declining at an overall rate of 8% per decade, starting in the third decade of life. The ability of the leg extensor muscles to develop power is of special relevance as it enables elderly people to accomplish daily tasks. The loss of leg extension power increases the risks of falls and limb disability. The age-related decline in muscle power is not prevented by rowing as shown by the lower bilateral dynamic leg extension power in older compared with young oarsmen (1675 vs. 2358 W) but older oarsmen possess a high power compared with older and young sedentary men (1261 and 1485 W, respectively). The parallel deterioration of skeletal muscular size and function is supported by a relationship between leg extension power and extensor muscle area (59–89 cm²; $r = 0.74$). Therefore, regular rowing has a profound effect in preventing muscle wasting and weakness.

Characteristics of elderly rowers

Masters rowing requires older participants of large body size, high level of aerobic capacity and muscular power as demonstrated by the observation in 32 older oarsmen (age, 59–73 years; height, 162–178 cm; body mass, 63–86 kg; body fat, 12–25%). A large body size provides an advantage to row 2000 m on an ergometer in that the performance (460–520 s) is related to body height ($r = 0.31$), body mass ($r = 0.60$) and fat free mass ($r = 0.78$; Fig. 10.3). The association of performance time with $\dot{V}O_{2max}$ (2.2–3.8 L·min⁻¹; $r = 0.71$) and $\dot{V}_{Emax}$ (79–151 L·min⁻¹; $r = 0.62$) suggests that a high level of cardiovascular and pulmonary function also has a role in the rowing performance of the elderly rower. Also, the

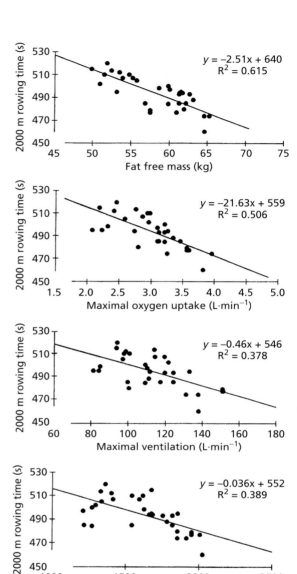

Fig. 10.3 Relationship between 2000 m rowing performance and fat free mass, maximal oxygen uptake and maximal ventilation in older men.

association of rowing performance time (470–520 s) with the area of leg extensor muscles (68–89 cm²; $r = 0.63$) and bilateral leg extension power (1271–2025 W; $r = 0.62$) indicates that both size and power of the leg extensor muscles are critical for Masters rowing performance. Thus, the physical require-

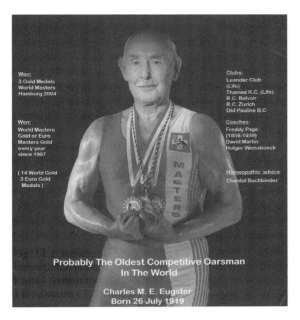

Fig. 10.4 Charles M.E. Eugster, born July 26, 1919: probably the oldest competitive oarsman in the world.

ments of elderly oarsmen are consistent with those observed in young counterparts (Fig. 10.4).

Benefit of rowing

Rowing contributes to proper body composition, aerobic fitness and healthy cardiovascular and skeletal muscular conditions and has preventive effects on indices for the development of coronary artery disease and type II diabetes. In addition, rowing has a low injury rate. Use of large muscle mass during combined arm and leg exercise allows for both cardiorespiratory and muscular training effects (Fig. 10.5).

Recommended reading

American College of Sports Medicine (1998) Exercise and physical activity for older adults. *Medicine and Science in Sports and Exercise* **30**, 992–1008.

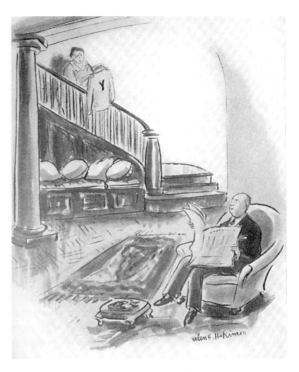

Fig. 10.5 "You aren't going to need the Yale crew sweater again, are you, Osgood?"

Blair, S.N. & Brodney, S. (1999) Effects of physical inactivity and obesity on morbidity and mortality: current evidence and research issues. *Medicine and Science in Sports and Exercise* **31**, S646–S662.

Drinkwater, B.L. (1994) Physical activity, fitness and osteoporosis. In: C. Bouchard, R.J. Shephard & T. Stephens, eds. *Physical Activity, Fitness, and Health, International Proceedings and Consensus Statement*. Human Kinetics Publishers, IL. pp. 724–736.

Fritsch, W. (2000) Rowing in daily life. In: W. Fritsch, ed. *Rowing*. Meyer & Meyer Sport Ltd, Oxford. pp. 148–183.

Pedersen, B.K. & Saltin, B. (2006) Evidence for prescribing exercise as therapy in chronic disease. *Scandinavian Journal of Medicine and Science in Sports* **16** (Suppl 1), 3–63.

Yoshiga, C.C. & Higuchi, M. (2003) Rowing performance of female and male rowers. *Scandinavian Journal of Medicine and Science in Sports* **13**, 317–321.

Chapter 11
Sports medicine

R. Budgett, D.M. Hettinga and J. Steinacker

Safety

Safety, as a form of preventive medicine, and fairness in training and competition are the two principal considerations addressed within the Fédération Internationale des Sociétés d'Aviron (FISA) regulations. For safety reasons, rowers are required to have a swimming certificate. In some countries a swimming test together with a capsize drill is performed in a pool to ensure that the rower is able to swim with his or her clothes for a minimum distance (e.g., 300 m). Singles, pairs and doubles may be more likely to capsize than larger boats, such as fours and eights, in which a capsize is more likely to occur at landing stages if participants do not use the correct procedure for getting in and out of the boat, in the event of a collision, or when letting go of the oar or scull handle(s). Tandem rigged fours (where the middle pair of rowers is rowing on the same side) are prone to rolling over when turning in poor conditions. However, as the intact capsized vessel provides flotation, by virtue of its sealed bow and stern compartments, rowers are advised not to attempt to swim to the shore. In the capsize drill, the rower is demonstrating his or her ability following capsize to release him or herself from the foot-stretchers, return the single sculls boat in the upright position and climb on it again. To enhance the release of the feet from the foot-stretchers and allow the rowers to get clear of the boat without using their hands in the event of capsize, FISA requires that the heels have restraints that are tight and short enough to

limit the heel rising above the lowest fixed point of the shoe. Such provision is controlled by an official (umpire) prior to launching. When officiating, the umpire stands upright in the launch and wears specific clothing (dark blue blazer, light blue shirt, FISA tie and gray trousers and, if worn, a dark blue hat). In wet weather, the umpire may wear a blue raincoat while, in very hot weather, he or she may officiate in shirtsleeves, with or without a tie. For sea rowing there is a limitation on how far from the shore rowing vessels can travel (e.g., in Denmark it is 2.5 km). Coxswains, umpires, coaches and launch personnel may be required to wear a flotation device.

Olympic rowing shells are also required to have a rubber ball fitted on their bow to absorb some of the impact of a collision. To minimize the likelihood of a collision, rowing courses are regulated by circulation rules where certain lanes are allocated to each traffic direction and at least one clear lane of water (13.5 m) is identified as a neutral lane between crews traveling in opposite directions (Fig. 11.1).

Violation of the traffic regulations, besides disqualification, can lead to serious accidents as was the case when a pair collided with a single scull in the 1992 Essen Regatta causing injuries to the sculler's leg that required five reconstructive surgeries and long hospitalization. In addition to the traffic regulations the rowers, while warming up or cooling down, shall not cross the finish line (in any direction) while boats from another race are finishing or follow a race over all or part of the course, even outside the buoyed area, when not taking part in a

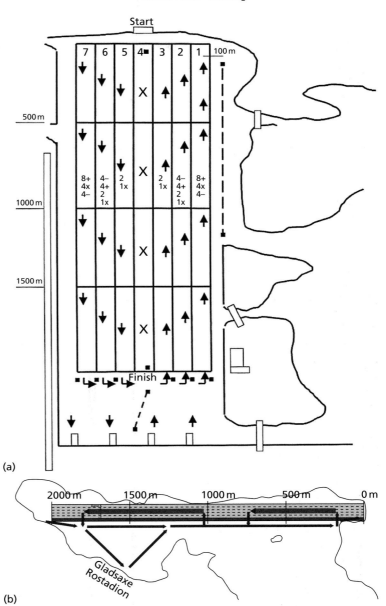

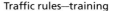

Fig. 11.1 Traffic regulations during training (a) and racing (b).

race. Also, crews should stop when competing crews approach their position.

Other safety measures regulate the construction of equipment. The opening of the coxswain's seat must be at least 70 cm long and it must be as wide as the boat for at least 50 cm. The edges of the oar and scull blades must have a minimum thickness of 5 and 3 mm, respectively, throughout. Boats constructed after January 1, 2007 must also show on a plaque placed in the boat whether the boat meets "FISA's Minimum Guidelines for the Safe Practice of Rowing": A boat when full of water with a crew of average weight equal to the design weight stated on the boat's production plaque, seated in the rowing position should float such that the top of the seat is a maximum of 5 cm below the static waterline.

Most Olympic rowing boats are coxless and the rower in the bow has the responsibility for steering with one foot-stretcher connected to a rudder in sweep boats. In sculling boats no rudder is provided and the rowers have to correct the direction by adjusting the power applied to each side. When rowing outside a proper race course, it is advised that a line of buoys is placed to separate the opposite traffic. Most often traffic to other vessels is prohibited in areas reserved for rowing. In sea rowing, however, where rowing and sailing boats meet, the vessel with the less ability to maneuver has the right of way and, as such, the rowing boat gives way to the sailing boat if they are in a collision course. The rowing boat has to choose the side of the sailing boat that is opposite to the direction of the wind (i.e., the side to which the sailing boat is leaning). If the sailing boat has to change its course, it has to move towards the direction of the wind. Motorboats have to respect rowing boats but the local traffic rules have to be followed and clear distance needs to be respected from the course of major vessels.

In the Victoria Falls Regatta in Zimbabwe, rowers share the course with hippopotami, elephants and crocodiles. Seated next to the umpire is a professional hunter to fend off any hippopotamus or crocodile that may stray too close to the competitors. The umpire also has the task of escorting rowers for each race to the start line. Very rarely, a hippo might upset, tip or bite a boat in half but incidences of direct attacks on humans are rare. In one occasion the course had to be altered when a hippopotamus decided to settle in.

During winter when the days are short and the water cold there are local rules regulating the times when rowing is allowed and it may be required that the boat is followed by a motorboat.

Rowing injuries

Rowing can be practiced into old age with great health benefits and the injury rate is similar to

swimming, or approximately 0.4 per thousand hours at the elite level. Although the injury rate may be higher among non-elite recreational rowers, when expressed as an hourly rate, it is still far less than other sports such as football (4 per thousand hours) or rugby (40 per thousand hours).

Low back pain is considered the most serious and significant injury but there is no evidence that the incidence of low back pain is any greater in rowers compared with athletes from other sports, or in people who do not participate in athletic events, because low back pain is so common in the general population.

In the last 20 years there has been an apparent increase in chest wall (rib) pain because of increased recognition and/or incidence. However, chest wall pain rarely causes more than a few weeks of missed training and is not considered as significant, or severe, as low back pain in rowers.

As many injuries are not caused by rowing but by weight training or other cross-training, especially running, caution is suggested in the interpretation of descriptive data as most research on rowers is anecdotal.

Overuse injuries

The majority of rowing injuries are caused by the repetitive rowing strokes and such forced contractions are concentrated in the major joints. Almost all muscle groups and joints are active at some point of the rowing stroke and any weaknesses, imbalances or tightness may predispose to an injury. The most commonly quoted problem is hamstring tightness and inflexibility.

Overuse injuries are more likely to occur with poor technique, poor flexibility, poor conditioning, imbalances, muscle weaknesses and faulty equipment.

Sculling, sweep oared rowing and ergometer (indoor) rowing are all similar types of exercise but they may predispose to different injuries. Coxes may also be injured, particularly suffering from anterior knee pain when steering from the stern of the boat. Overuse injuries are more common in female than male rowers. In women, chest wall injuries are slightly more common than low back pain, which is more common than tenosynovitis of the wrist extensors. In men, low back pain is more common than tenosynovitis of the wrist, which is more common than chest wall pain.

Low back pain

There is no evidence that the incidence of low back pain is increasing, or that the incidence of very severe career-ending back pain is increasing despite concerns that increases in training volume and changes in equipment, including increased use of rowing ergometers, might cause this. In common with ex-Olympic weightlifters, there is a lower incidence of back pain in ex-rowers than in the general population. This may be a result of selection bias because an injury-free back is needed to reach the elite level of both sports, but it is likely that back strength protects against low back pain.

A history of low back pain is not a contraindication to rowing. Many individuals will benefit from a rowing program and there is no more time lost out of the boat by rowers with a previous history of back injury than those with no previous history. Of injuries to rowers, 25–50% affect the low back. In some studies, 50% of these injuries are brought about by weight training, although only 10% of an elite rower's training time is spent weight training. The flexion and extension movement in rowing may be protective and helps rehabilitate an injured back, but this potential benefit is lost with the twisting motion of sweep oared rowing. In Britain, the Amateur Rowing Association does not allow children under 16 to race in sweep oared boats. They are restricted to sculling, and weight training is discouraged until bone maturity is reached.

Tight and weak hamstrings may predispose to lower back pain by reducing the normal anterior rotation of the pelvis and forcing an increased lumbar kyphosis. Weak or asymmetric hamstrings and hip flexors can also contribute. As a rower fatigues through a long training session, the range of movement of the lumbar spine increases from 75 to 90% of maximum. It is suggested that the increased torque when intervertebral disks are fully hydrated and at their largest in the early morning may contribute as many rowers train at this time.

Poor adherence to a stretching program of the hamstrings, gluteal and hip flexors is associated with an increased injury rate. The strength of these muscles and those supporting core stability are important. Maintaining intra-abdominal pressure helps stabilize the spine, reducing sheer forces between lumbar vertebrae. It is possible that inspiratory muscle training and expiration through the drive phase of the stroke can help.

Most low back pain in rowers is brought about by disk injury, particularly annular tear with or without prolapse, which may occasionally cause significant plural irritation and sciatica. Symptomatic disk injury confirmed by magnetic resonance imaging (MRI) scanning normally takes 3 months to fully resolve but, at the end of this time, the vast majority are back in full training and competition. Treatment involves relative rest, physiotherapy and medical interventions such as anti-inflammatory drugs, injections (epidural) and, rarely, surgery.

Other causes of low back pain are rare but include facet joint strain and spondylolysis. Such states tend to cause pain on extension and are normally secondary to inappropriate or poor quality weight training. Sacroiliac joint dysfunction may also occur, normally caused by land training.

Chest wall pain

Rib stress fractures are the most significant cause of chest wall pain in rowers and there has been an increase in the diagnosis of this problem in the last 20 years. The pain is felt in the anterolateral chest wall and can be pinpointed by the rower. This localization normally corresponds with the objective signs and clinical findings. Once a bony callus starts to form after 4–7 days, the lesion can be easily seen on ultrasound, isotope bone scans or computed tomography (CT) scans. X-ray is unlikely to show any abnormality (if ever) until healing is well advanced.

Rib stress fractures are most likely to occur whenever there is a change in training. This may be an increase in volume or intensity, a change of side in a sweep oared rower, or a change in training to or from sculling, rowing and land ergometer training.

The etiology of rib stress is controversial but probably involves compressive forces on the ribs rather than a traction effect from the serratus anterior. The serratus anterior may be involved in that if it fatigues, there is a loss of resistance to the compressive forces caused by an increase in abdominal pressure. The serratus anterior contracts maximally when the shoulder is retracted at the finish and it is forced to contract eccentrically, which means that the force developed is ~20% higher than during a shortening contraction. The prevalence of chest wall injuries in women may be related to their reduced ability, compared with men, to increase connective tissue with training. There is uncertainty regarding the cause of rib stress fractures in rowers and so no clear or agreed prevention strategy. The pathology and prevention of rib stress fractures will be one of the most useful areas of research in rowing injuries. Recovery is normally quicker than would be expected in other stress fractures, with a return to rowing after 2–4 weeks. Only a small minority take more than 5 weeks to return to full training.

The differential diagnosis of chest wall pain in rowers includes intercostal muscle strains, costochondritis or costal vertebral joints subluxation. These causes should be distinguished with a good history and careful examination. Nevertheless, if there is doubt about the diagnosis, investigation with ultrasound or isotope bone scan is helpful.

Wrist and forearm pain

Tenosynovitis, inflammation of the tendon and its enveloping sheath, of the wrist extensors is a common injury well known to all rowers. So-called "teno" is easy to recognize by pain, swelling and grating proximal to the wrist. Intersection syndrome is most common, affecting extensor carpi radialis longus and brevis but may also be related to friction between abductor pollicis longus and extensor pollicis brevis, so-called de Quervain's tenosynovitis. These muscles are located in the forearm and their tendons travel across the wrist (through a "tunnel" termed the first dorsal compartment) on the thumb side to produce movement of the thumb. The condition is 10 times more common in women, more often arises in the dominant hand and usually occurs between the ages of 35 and 55. The diagnosis is easy by palpating a "snowball" feeling over the tendons when the thumb is moving.

Compartment syndrome of the forearm is a differential diagnosis and can be diagnosed with pressure studies. The whole compartment is tight and painful and there is no localized swelling and grating.

Forearm pain is normally related to training errors, particularly a sudden increase or change in training, or gripping the oar handle too tightly. Equipment may contribute if the handle is too small and the gate too tight so that feathering is forceful. Conditions may also contribute. In rough water an athlete will grip the oar handle tightly. The symptoms can appear surprisingly suddenly through one outing and then persist for many weeks.

Treatment consists of relative rest, often using splints, physiotherapy modalities and local anti-inflammatory treatment, including ice, can help. Injection of corticosteroid is sometimes used and in urgent or refractory cases surgical decompression is effective. If symptoms improve, adding gentle stretching exercises (stretch the thumb into the palm) can prevent recurrent inflammation.

Other injuries

Anterior knee pain is rare except for coxes or after heavy cross-training such as running or weight training. Rowing is good treatment for any athlete with anterior knee pain, helping to build up the vastus medialis, and optimize tracking of the patella. There is minimal eccentric loading.

Coxes sitting in the stern of the boat with knees drawn up, resisting the acceleration and deceleration with each stroke, report a much higher incidence of anterior knee pain than the rowers.

Blisters and abrasions are very common. These are generally minor and accepted as part of rowing, particularly at the beginning of the season, when hands may have softened. The constant exposure to water dries and hardens the skin. As a result a new blister may be created below the first and, eventually, become infected (Fig. 11.2).

Abrasions commonly occur to the calves from the slide bed digging into the back of the athlete's leg. Abrasions may also occur on the knuckles in scullers as the left hand passes over the right. These injuries are generally of no significance unless there is an infection. Reports of blood poisoning from such infections have been noted, thus infections sometimes need to be treated with antibiotics. Rowers

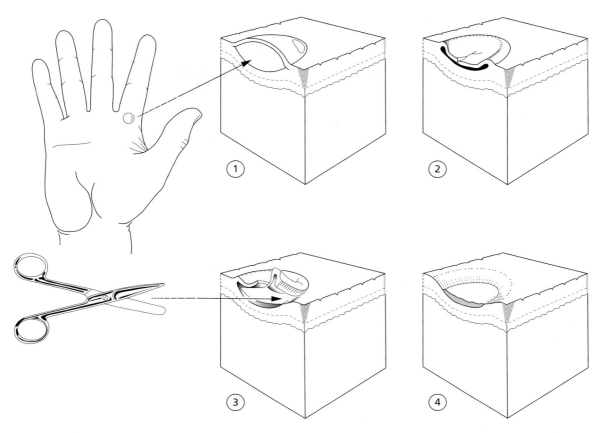

Fig. 11.2 Making sure that there is no hard skin developing at the edge of a blister. It is important that the ridge of hard skin is cut at a 45° angle. © Skanning 1989.

must keep the wounds clean, carefully pare down calluses and avoid using gloves which, as well as reducing blade control and proprioception, can also make friction blisters worse.

Water-borne diseases

The water we row upon is not always as clean and certainly is not pure enough to be swallowed. There are risks to health associated with water-based activities, which arise from the microbiologic or chemical quality of the water itself and of its immediate environment. The use of inland waters can never be risk free and it is essential that rowers are aware of the risks present.

Weill's disease — leptospirosis

The risk of contracting leptospirosis from recreational water is small; however, the serious nature of the disease is such that rowers must be aware of the dangers and should take the following simple precautions to reduce the risk of infection:
• Cuts and abrasions (including blisters) should be covered with waterproof dressings
• When paddling in the water (launching the boat), footwear should be worn to avoid cuts and protect feet
• After contact with the water rowers should shower and wash hands thoroughly before eating and drinking
If flu-like symptoms develop shortly after contact

with the water (1–3 weeks) then your doctor should be contacted and advised of the circumstances of exposure.

Blue–green algae — Cynobacteria

Cynobacteria are commonly found in fresh and brackish water during mid to late summer. In favorable stable conditions, blooms may form. Algal scums accumulate downwind on the surface of lakes and slow-moving water. Toxins produced by large blooms have caused the death of sheep and dogs, and skin and other disorders in humans, although no particular illness has been identified that can be linked with blue–green algae.

As precautions rowers should:
• Avoid immersion or contact with water affected by algal scum
• Minimize contact with water by wearing close-fitting clothing
• After any contact all equipment should be washed to avoid contact with residual scum
• All clothing should be washed and thoroughly dried
• Shower after contact with the water

Summary

Rowing is safer than most other Olympic sports. Low back pain, rib pain and tenosynovitis are the most common overuse injuries. Acute traumatic injuries are very rare.

Prevention includes optimizing training with adequate periodization and recovery. Great care when changing the volume, intensity and type of training and correctly using cross-training and conditioning with particular care when weight training. Weight training must be properly supervised and the maximum weight a rower should lift in training is the weight at which they can continue to maintain lifting technique. Good core stability, stretching after training and strengthening of antagonist muscles also help to prevent injuries. With appropriate training and prevention strategies rowing is a sport that most individuals should be able to enjoy from early teens, through retirement and beyond.

Travel

Rowers suffer similar problems to anyone traveling long distances, namely travel fatigue and jet-lag, and it is important to minimize these if training and performance are to be maintained. Preparation should start long before departure to make sure that the journey itself is as stress free as possible. The food and drink offered on aircrafts is often inadequate for rowers in hard training, so they should bring their own in sealed containers to the extent allowed by the increasing safety precautions of air carriers. Essentials for training or competition should be kept in hand luggage.

Jet-lag is the disruption of normal circadian rhythms as they adjust to a new time zone. Many bodily functions fluctuate over a 24 h period. Most obvious is sleep and waking but the kidneys, gut and endocrine system all follow a 24 h cycle and adjust to changing time zones at different speeds, contributing to the symptoms of fatigue, loss of concentration, loss of appetite, headache, dizziness and nausea.

Standard advice is to allow 1 day of adjustment per hour time difference. It may be possible to adjust more quickly traveling west. During this time rowers are advised to reduce both the intensity and volume of training. Strategies to reduce jet-lag should be discussed with team support staff or experts. It is important to adjust watches, clocks and all activities as soon as possible to the new time zone (right from the start of the journey). Rowers should avoid sleeping during the day after arrival and if they have to sleep should limit this to 1 h maximum sleep time. Waking and meals should all be at the appropriate time for the new time zone with appropriate food for the meal. The strongest influence on circadian rhythms is light. Rowers should expose themselves to daylight, or at least bright artificial light, at the correct time alternating with darkness at night time, to help reset the body clock. When traveling westwards, it may be helpful to train at midday to early evening and when travelling eastwards to train in the early evening, exposing the body to activity and light forcing wakefulness at a time when the rower is feeling sleepy.

Drugs have been used to try to help speed adjustment or to ease the symptoms of jet-lag. Melatonin is not recommended for routine use, because it is unlicensed in most countries and so may be of poor quality. Melatonin may be contaminated, which could have implications for anti-doping tests and has unpredictable effects, causing no sleepiness in some individuals and prolonged drowsiness in others. Sleeping pills such as temazepam or zopiclone (shorter acting) should not be used on the flight because they may contribute to immobility and the risk of deep vein thrombosis (DVT). Although sleeping pills effectively promote sleep, there is reduced rapid eye movement (REM) sleep, so the regenerative power of sleeping is less effective. Such medication is addictive and should never be used for more than a week. Nevertheless, rowers and teams traveling abroad often do use sleeping pills for two or three nights after arrival if any members are unable to sleep. It is recommended to take aspirin (75 mg·day^{-1}) for 1 week prior to air travel in order to prevent the development of DVT.

When travelling the team should remember to check immunizations required in good time, as it may take at least a month to complete a protective course. They should also check whether malarial tablets are needed. Further detailed advice on traveling can be found through the World Health Organization (www.who.int) and individual departments of health in most countries.

Diabetes

Like asthma, diabetes may occur in rowers of all standards including Olympic Champions, as in, most famously, Sir Steven Redgrave, five times Olympic gold medallist (see Fig. 1.10). Diabetes is caused by a reduction in insulin production (type I) and/or a reduced sensitivity of the body's cells to insulin (type II). It is a complex and important disease, more common with the western lifestyle and diet, particularly in the overweight. The lack of insulin or its lack of effect produce high sugar levels in the blood and so in urine and can lead to many complications over time including heart disease,

blindness and kidney failure. With good sugar control the risk of these complications can be greatly reduced. Fast-acting insulin given four or more times a day has enabled diabetics to meet their needs for insulin far more effectively and has also been a great help to athletes with diabetes. Diabetics are now able to live a normal life, with no limitation on their intake of carbohydrates (vital for sports performance) and are encouraged to eat the same healthy diet (low in fat, high in carbohydrates) as the rest of the population. Endurance exercise such as rowing is beneficial to diabetics as the sensitivity of the body cells to insulin is increased and so blood sugar control is easier and the requirement for insulin reduced. Diabetic rowers training 4 h per day sometimes need no insulin through periods of particularly hard exercise and can fine tune and control their blood sugar levels by monitoring, carbohydrate intake and insulin injections as needed. It is important that hard exercising rowers get specialist advice on control of their diabetes so as to avoid hypoglycemia (sugar levels falling too low), which is a risk if they do not take enough carbohydrate and/or use too much insulin and/or use up all carbohydrate stores by exercise. High blood sugar is also seen in cases when prednisolone is taken.

Asthma

Asthma and exercise-induced asthma can affect rowers of any standard from recreational to Olympic gold medallists. Symptoms can be controlled very effectively with medication, so it is important to identify and treat asthmatics properly. The classic symptoms are cough, wheeze, shortness of breath and a tight chest after and sometimes during exercise. This is association with airway obstruction and a drop in forced expiratory flow in 1 s (FEV_1). Most asthmatics will react to exercise, particularly in cold dry air but some only ever get symptoms as a result of exercise. Even in these rowers, there is usually some underlying airway inflammation and frequently their symptoms will be worse in association with colds, high pollen count or pollution. There may be a personal history of eczema or hayfever (atopy) or a family history of atopy. In some studies up to 50% of rowers reacted to cold dry air but the proven prevalence in fully investigated Olympic rowing squads is approximately 20%.

Diagnosis of exercise-induced asthma (EIA) involves challenge testing, to see if a stimulus reduces the expiratory flow, measured as FEV_1, significantly. The IOC has a threshold of 10% fall in FEV_1 as proof of diagnosis — otherwise the athlete is not allowed to use the medication. The challenge may be exercise in the laboratory (where the environment can be controlled) on a rowing machine or another ergometer. The test may be in the sporting environment, although symptoms may not be precipitated if it is a warm humid day. Eucapnic voluntary hyperpnea (EVH) test is a very sensitive and specific challenge reproducing the drying effect of exercise. However, it does require expensive equipment and is not universally available. Inhaled mannitol may be an easier and cheaper challenge but the EVH test is preferred by the IOC. Methacholine has been used to challenge the airways but is not used in the diagnosis of EIA.

Treatment is important because, left untreated, the underlying inflammation will slowly worsen. Precipitating factors should be avoided as much as possible. Rowers may find that after an attack there is a so-called refractory period when further attacks are unlikely. However, this is not a good way to control asthma. Salbutamol and terbutaline are very effective in controlling symptoms when taken approximately 15 min before exercise. They may produce tremor, rapid heart beat (tachycardia) and, if used regularly without preventative treatment, the underlying asthma will worsen. Anticholinergics such as ipratropium or tiotropium (longer acting) may have a role. The main stay of treatment is inhaled corticosteroids such as beclometasone or fluticasone. These are most effective when used in combination with a long-acting β_2-agonist such as salmeterol or formoterol. Other treatments for asthma are leukotriene receptor antagonists and sodium cromoglycate, but these are probably less effective in most rowers.

It is important to distinguish asthma, including EIA, from other causes of shortness of breath with exercise. These may include vocal chord dysfunction causing stridor with restriction of inhalation rather than restriction of exhalation as is seen in asthma. Reassurance, psychologic strategies and respiratory muscle training may help and there is sometimes an element of hyperventilation. Rowers should beware of herbal supplements, which are unlikely to be effective and may contain prohibited substances such as oral prednisolone not detailed on the label. Although there is no scientific evidence to confirm that inhaled β_2-agonists enhance performance in the dosage required to inhibit EIA, they are prohibited in the World Anti-Doping Agency (WADA) list and require an Abbreviated Therapeutic Use Exemption (ATUE). All inhaled corticosteroids also require an ATUE.

Coughing after intense exercise is not a sign of asthma but a normal response to increased lung fluid and disappears as the fluid returns to normal.

Health assessments in rowers

Substitutions

In the case of illness of, or injury to, a member of a crew before the first heat, a substitution may be made if a medical certificate is provided and if the change is approved by the Sports Medicine Commission of FISA. The replaced rower may compete at any point during the competition on production of a further medical certificate. Not more than half of the rowers in a crew (plus the coxswain, if applicable) may be changed. No substitution may be made of a single sculler.

Screening

Screening of athletes is controversial and not routinely cost effective. Nevertheless, preparticipation medicals are commonly completed and there are good arguments for profiling athletes and performing a basic medical check. The IOC now recommends cardiac screening with a questionnaire and electrocardiogram (ECG). Others recommend an echocardiogram is included but it is unclear what level of participation warrants this screening.

Profiling should include a history of any previous injuries because previous injury is the best predictor of any subsequent injury. A history of serious illness, especially epilepsy, asthma and any suspicion of syncope (collapse) should be taken. A careful medication and supplement history is important, particularly to make sure that no prohibited substances are being taken inadvertently and to check whether any Therapeutic Use Exemptions (TUEs) or ATUEs are needed. A family history, particularly of collapse or death before the age of 50, is important.

The focus of any physical examination should be on the factors reported in the history. A prevention program can then be put in place by the medical team, focusing on any previous injuries and also on common injuries in rowers such as low back pain. Most squads routinely prescribe a program of core stability and stretching, particularly of the hamstrings, to help prevent back pain. Preparticipation medicals are rarely necessary in recreational rowing and should not restrict access to the sport. Rowing is possible for most people whatever their disability with appropriate regulations to restrict participation to, for instance, land training in cases of uncontrolled epilepsy or in later pregnancy.

Preparticipation tests are performed regularly in Italy and France. There are reports of sudden death in rowing although it appears less frequently in rowing than in other sports and most often related to non-cardiac death. There is a recent report of a German lightweight rower who died, probably from dehydration, while a US rower died after crossing the finish line. It is known that fat deposits have been found in the wall of the right atrium of the heart in some people who become ill in association with exercise. Also, there have been a number of cases with skin infections resulting from *Staphylococcus aureus* and it is recommended to wipe ergometers (seat and handle) with alcohol before use. In some areas wasps are a problem at the end of the season and antihistamine tablets, with or without sedating effect, are recommended to be available for immediate use. Also, it is advised that rowers check their bottles for wasps before drinking.

Hyperthermia

Rowing training and regattas often take place in the warmer season of the year and therefore rowers are exposed to warm climates. These climates impose a health risk on rowers and in the case of regattas, also on visitors. Organizers should be prepared to evaluate the potential risks and take precautions. For the resting or exercising human, the net energy balance between heat production and heat loss determines body core temperature (Tc), which is related to well-being and athletic performance.

The body temperature is the balance between heat production and heat loss from the skin and the airways. Resting metabolic rate is increased with exercise and stress while about 75% of the whole metabolism during exercise produces heat instead of mechanical work. Heat loss consists of *conduction* (direct contact with air, water and other materials), *convection* (motion of air or liquids across the heated skin), *radiation* (infrared rays transport heat) and *evaporation/sweating* as fluid evaporates, heat is lost.

Clothing significantly influences heat loss. The heat insulation of the fabric and the moisture permeability are important and how these change with wind, body motion or both. Heat insulation is high in wool and similar textiles. Modern sport fabrics have moderate heat insulation and provide good cooling through high moisture permeability. Much rain gear has low moisture permeability and limits heat exchange significantly, because the body is insulated by the saturated air between skin and garment. When a rain garment enables some kind of air pumping over the skin during the exercise, additional heat may be lost which is beneficial. Airtight clothing contributes to the number of heat-related disorders and some deaths in athletes. Some water-tight fabrics enable exchange of some quantities of moisture and increase thermal comfort.

The environmental factors that contribute to heat balance of the body are ambient air temperature, wind velocity, relative air humidity and mean radiant temperature (from radiation; sun, car, walls). Commonly, the environmental influences are represented by measurement of air temperature. However, the net energy balance is determined mainly by the heat exchange of the skin and by breathing. Wind velocity determines the heat convection and the heat loss by sweating. The relative air humidity determines mainly the effects of sweating, as with high humidity the effect of sweating may be severely diminished. Conditions with high air humidity

Table 11.1 Temperature effects of environmental factors for a lightweight rower exercising in rain gear at low rowing speed in the open sun.

Ambient temperature	20.0°C (68°F)	
Air humidity	+0.5°C (1°F)	For each extra 20% air humidity
Radiation effect	+7.0°C (13°F)	Sunny sky
Clothing	+6.7°C (12°F)	Insulation effect of the rain gear
Physical exercise	+24.0°C (43°F)	1506 kJ·h^{-1} during training
Air convection	−5.6°C (10°F)	"Wind" benefit from rowing
Equivalent air temperature	55.4°C (132°F)	

Table 11.2 Increase in body core temperature in relation to oxygen uptake.

% $\dot{V}O_{2max}$	Increase in body core temperature
50	1.2°C
70	2.0°C
80	2.5°C
90	3.2°C

impose high risk for thermal regulation. Radiation is represented by mean radiant temperature; it is high with a sunny sky and low in cloudy conditions. Radiation is also present in overheated cars and rooms. Thus, in rowing, body temperature is highly dependent on weather conditions (Table 11.1).

The term "wet bulb globe temperature" (WBGT) is commonly used to quantify environmental heat stress. WBGT is often used for calculation of the thermal risk of a given condition and describes the energy balance of a wet dark standard body at the given climate of an area. Actual WBGT values may be obtained from any meteorology station and from calculators on the Internet (www.pphsa.on.ca/OccHealth/HeatStress/WBGT_Calc.htm).

Skin temperature and heat balance

Skin temperature is closely related to heat loss. Uncovered skin is effective in losing heat by convection, radiation and sweating as explained above. That is only the case if circulation is maintained. When water losses lead to decreased water content of the body (hypohydration), this will lead to a paradoxically cold, wet skin because of peripheral vasoconstriction and (reduced) sweat production. This highlights the importance of continuous replacement of water loss (rehydration) as a precaution measure.

As a rule of thumb, a decrease of body water content of 5% will increase body core temperature by 1–1.3°C mainly by impairing skin blood flow.

Body temperature

Small increases in muscle temperature can make muscles' energy systems more efficient, which is used in the warming up. In exercising muscles, temperature may reach 42°C (107.6°F). Body core temperature can exceed 40°C (104°F) during exercise. Performance decreases when body core temperatures rise above 40°C which can affect the nervous system and reduce the ability to unload excess heat. With increasing temperatures rapidly central nervous symptoms and serious brain damage can occur. Temperatures above 44°C (111°F) can not be sustained without serious damage.

Effects of physical training and competition

The metabolic effect of exercise is important for temperature control because work efficiency is only ~20% for rowing, which means that the remaining 80% has to dissipate as heat. This is obviously no problem in cold environments but in warm climates body core temperature may increase beyond the normal increase with exercise intensity (Table 11.2). This exercise-induced amount of heat is then transported by the blood flow to the lungs where the inspired air is humidified and warmed up. Therefore, the lungs are the first heat exchanging organ but of limited capacity. The lungs have good heat exchange efficiency at low ambient temperatures and dry air, but when the ambient temperature rises near body temperature and the air is more water saturated the efficiency decreases.

The skin has a major role in heat exchange with the environment. However, the skin function is totally dependent on an intact circulation. With increasing heat production, a larger portion of cardiac output has to be directed to the skin for heat exchange. This means that maximum performance may be limited in hot climates because of temperature regulation.

After exercise and racing, the wind convection is decreased and particularly after races, a high amount of heat has to be unloaded. This puts an additional burden to the already stressed central nervous system and can lead in some case to collapse, loss of consciousness and, if untreated, to fatality. Immediate after racing, rowers will tend to recover faster if they do not lie down and move slowly, if they do not relax too much (lose central control), if they cool themselves with water and rehydrate quickly.

At high ambient temperatures, additional cooling with water is a very good strategy to increase heat exchange through the skin because water has a far better heat capacity than air.

Sweating and body fluid losses

The water losses during exercise at 60% of $\dot{V}O_{2max}$ at 21°C (70°F) air temperature can be estimated as $1 L \cdot h^{-1}$ by sweating and $0.1–0.2 L \cdot h^{-1}$ by breathing. Additionally, approximately 0.5 g sodium chloride and other minerals (potassium, calcium and magnesium) are lost with sweat (Table 11.3) and approximately 50 mg potassium is lost with urine. These water and salt losses increase in high ambient temperature and decrease with acclimatization. In addition, iron is lost by sweating and can eventually lead to iron deficiency anemia.

Water loss leads to a decrease in body water content, plasma and blood volume. A decrease of

more than 2% in plasma volume leads to a decrease in physical performance. Two-thirds of the body weight is roughly total body water content. The weight changes during dehydration can be attributed mainly to water losses, not more than approximately 20% can be contributed to losses in substrates such as glycogen, glucose, proteins and fat. The effects of decreased plasma and blood volume lead to decreased skin blood flow and impaired thermoregulation as described above. This can be counter-regulated by the kidneys, which reabsorb water and increase the osmolality of the urine.

In a study in German lightweight rowers, when ambient temperature increased from 18 to 28°C (64.4–82.4°F), hematocrit increased by 5% and plasma volume decreased by 10% within days. In this range performance and health are clearly challenged.

The effects of heat-induced water loss can be summarized as follows:
1 High volumes of sweat
2 Decreased plasma and blood volume
3 Loss of minerals and electrolytes (sodium chloride, potassium, magnesium)
4 Release of aldosterone and antidiuretic hormone (ADH) and water reabsorption in kidneys
5 Increased osmolality of the urine

Weighing is a good and simple measure of water loss. Urine osmolality can be assessed visually (light color: low osmolality, no problem; dark: high osmolality, water deficit) and measured with urine sticks. Rehydration can be based on urine osmolality and a simple estimation is urine volume, which should be higher than $2 L \cdot day^{-1}$. When exposed to a hot climate, the loss of salt through sweating is a consideration and rowers may be at risk of miner's cramps (water poisoning). It is advised that in a hot environment salt tablets are provided with at least one daily meal.

In some teams, hematocrit is used as a measure of hydration status. Hematocrit is the cell part of blood and is estimated by centrifugation. The hematocrit should be lower than 50%, optimum levels are considered between 42% and 48%. Hematocrit is influenced by body position during sampling and it requires capillary blood sampling and a centrifuge.

Table 11.3 Electrolyte concentrations in sweat (osmolality 150 mmol·kg^{-1}).

	Concentration	
	mg·L^{-1}	mmol·L^{-1}
Na$^+$	413–1091	18.0–47.5
Cl$^-$	533–1495	15.0–42.2
K$^+$	121–255	3.1–6.5
Mg^{2+}	4–34	0.2–1.4
Ca^{2+}	85–109	2.1–2.7

Acclimatization

The most important prevention strategy is heat acclimatization which can improve performance quite dramatically so that acclimated subjects can easily complete exercise in the heat, which earlier was difficult or impossible to achieve.

The minimum time for heat acclimatization for unacclimatized athletes is 3 days, while total heat acclimatization is achieved after 14–21 days. This has to be taken into account when preparing in cold climates for competitions in warm conditions. Heat acclimatization and heat tolerance are different for individuals and there appears to be a learning effect so that previous exposure to a warm climate makes a subsequent exposure more tolerable.

Hypothermia

Hypothermia occurs when the whole of the body has been chilled to much lower than 35°C. The following are the most usual symptoms and signs of hypothermia, but not all may be present.
• Unexpected and unreasonable behavior possibly accompanied by complaints of coldness and tiredness
• Physical and mental lethargy with failure to understand a question or orders
• Slurring of speech
• Violent outburst of unexpected energy and violent language, becoming uncooperative
• Failure of, or abnormality in vision
• Twitching
• Lack of motor control, unsteadiness and complaining of numbness and cramps
• General shock with pallor and blueness of lips and nails
• Slow weak heart rate, wheezing and coughing

Avoidance must be the first consideration at all times. Layers of clothing are more effective than one warm garment. The head is a major source of heat loss and to reduce this loss some sort of head gear is recommended. Exposed arms legs and head heighten the risk. Sudden immersion in cold water can have a shock effect, which can disrupt normal breathing and provoke hyperventilation which eliminates carbon dioxide in the expired air and reduces cerebral blood flow with detrimental effect on cerebral oxygenation, reducing even a proficient swimmer to incompetence. Confusion and an inability to respond to simple instructions become evident. Thus, it is advised to try to control breathing and minimize hyperventilation. When a person has fallen into cold water their body loses heat rapidly. Even in a normal summer, the water temperature is rarely sufficient to avoid hypothermic conditions. To reduce heat loss it is advised to keep clothes on except for heavy coats or boots, which may drag the person down.

Anti-doping

The IOC introduced the first anti-doping regulations in the late 1960s. Initially, anabolic agents and stimulants were prohibited. The prohibited list now covers a much wider variety of drugs and the IOC handed over responsibility to WADA in 2004. Substances or methods that may improve performance but are a danger to health, or against the spirit of sport, may be considered for inclusion on the prohibited list.

Much time and effort has been spent educating rowers throughout the world on the importance of fair competition without using prohibited substances or methods. In rowing there are far fewer positive results than in many other Olympic sports but there is still concern regarding anabolic agents, stimulants and erythropoietin (EPO) or other methods of enhancing oxygen transfer. Recently, WADA suggested that the use of hypoxic tents violates the spirit of sport and therefore should be included on the list of banned substances but that is still debated.

At present FISA does not advocate blood sampling for the assessment of hematocrit level in rowers and therefore the no-start limit of 50% is not used as in cycling. The reason for this decision is that screening does not support widespread abuse of blood-enhancing products such as EPO or autologous blood transfusion. As blood hemoglobin is normally distributed, it remains a problem that some individuals consistently show high values (Fig. 11.3).

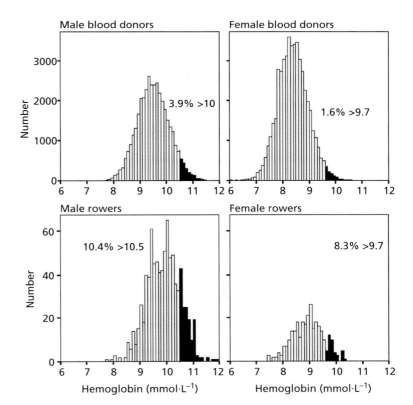

Fig. 11.3 Forearm venous hemoglobin concentration in 85,846 Danish blood donors and 1459 Danish elite rowers. A total of 3.9% of the male and 1.6% of the female blood donors as well as 10.4% of the rowers had blood hemoglobin above the no-start limit (P. Johansson and K. Jensen, the HS blood bank and the University of Southern Denmark).

Also, distribution of hemoglobin is affected by variation in plasma volume, drinking and even positioning of the athlete. Furthermore, performance is related to total hemoglobin rather than to the hemoglobin concentration in blood as in hematosis. For all these reasons it would be more relevant to establish blood doping criteria based on determination of total hemoglobin than on the hemoglobin concentration or hematocrit.

The current doping list (2007, www.wada-ama. org) covers anabolic agents such as testosterone and stanozolol; anti-oestrogenic agents such as tamoxifen; β_2-agonists such as salbutamol, although some of these are permitted by inhalation if an ATUE form has been submitted; cannabinoids (in competition only); diuretics and other masking agents such as probenecid. Corticosteroids (in competition only) such as beclometasone and hydrocortisone are prohibited when administered orally, rectally or by intravenous or intramuscular injection. Inhalation and local injection of corticosteroids is prohibited unless an ATUE form has

been submitted. Hormones and related substances such as EPO and growth hormone; narcotics (in competition) such as morphine; stimulants (in competition only) such as cocaine and ephedrine. Alcohol and beta-blockers are prohibited in particular sports such as shooting. Prohibited methods are enhancement of oxygen transfer, classically blood doping; chemical and physical manipulation such as trying to interfere with the urine sample, and gene doping (the non-therapeutic use of genetic elements).

Testing is carried out by national anti-doping organizations, national and international federations, WADA, the IOC and the International Paralympic Committee (IPC). Testing is carried out both in and out of competition with increasing emphasis on out of competition testing, using both urine and blood. The blood is used to identify athletes whose profile may be a result of abuse. The introduction of a whereabouts system so that athletes can be tested at any time has further enhanced the deterrent effect of anti-doping programs.

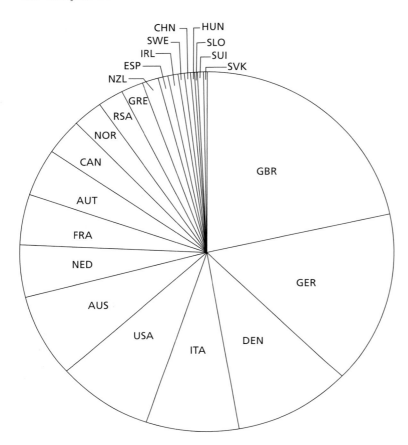

Fig. 11.4 Therapeutic use exemptions (TUEs) submitted in 2005.

A TUE can be granted by any anti-doping agency if an appropriate committee feels that the prohibited substance or method is medically essential, there is no reasonable alternative available and it is unlikely to enhance performance. Asthma inhalers (the β_2-agonists, salbutamol, terbutaline, salmeterol and formoterol, and all corticosteroids) just need notification in the form of an ATUE, but the β_2-agonists need proof of diagnosis submitted to the IOC for the Olympic Games. FISA currently requires a statement of what diagnostics tests have been used but no proof of results. Cortisone injections need an ATUE, TUE or no TUE at all depending on the route. This has changed yearly for the last 3 years with details in the WADA Prohibited List. In 2007, topical corticosteroids do not require any notification. This includes skin creams, eye drops, ear drops, nose sprays and iontophoresis. Corticosteroids given by inhalation or a local injection (not into the muscle) need an ATUE and systemic corticosteroids (oral,

muscular injection or rectal) need a full TUE. The number of TUEs sent to FISA each year is about 300–400. Some countries have a high notification rate than others (Fig. 11.4).

Although anti-doping appears to concentrate on elite rowers, the Master athletes also need some attention. Because 1500 out of 3000 Master athletes have submitted a TUE or ATUE, as many Masters take medications for high blood pressure, atrial fibrillation, high cholesterol, diuretics, it is concerning that such practice may mask the use of doping.

Doping in spinal cord injured rowers

Adaptive rowers, as all other rowers, are subject to the anti-doping regulations as issued by WADA and FISA. However, the IPC has issued an additional regulation, which applies to athletes with high thoracic or cervical spinal cord lesions. As a result of an impaired autonomic nervous system, these athletes can enhance their performance by a self-induced increase in blood pressure, known as boosting. However, there are considerable medical risks associated with this technique, which is why the IPC has banned boosting on medical safety grounds.

A lesion in the spinal cord above the sixth thoracic vertebra leads to an impaired sympathetic outflow, which is particularly noticeable in tetraplegics. In these individuals a nociceptive stimulus below the level of the spinal cord injury — such as an extended bladder or bowel, an injury to the body below the level of lesion or an infection — can trigger an abnormal sympathetic reflex. The body responds to such a stimulus by vasoconstriction below the level of the lesion resulting in a massive increase in peripheral resistance. The consequent increase in blood pressure is detected by the baroreceptors, but the necessary action to this hypertension is impaired. Although the heart responds by lowering the heart rate, the spinal lesion prevents sympathetic signals from controlling the peripheral circulation. The response, therefore, is inadequate and the blood pressure remains high, while heart rate is low. This phenomenon is known as autonomic dysreflexia (AD) and can be a life-threatening condition because the elevated blood pressure increases the risk for seizures, cerebral hemorrhage, cardiac problems and even death.

Symptoms of AD include headache, piloerection, sweating and generally feeling unwell. In most cases these symptoms disappear quickly when the nociceptive stimulus is taken away; however, in severe cases urgent medical intervention is required. Most individuals susceptible to AD carry nifedepine with them and this should be taken when severe symptoms occur.

Individuals with a lesion above T6 can trigger an AD response by, for example, blocking the catheter, inflicting a wound or sitting on the scrotum. The resulting increase in blood pressure can compensate for the low cardiac output seen in many persons with high spinal lesions. Because of an absent muscle pump, blood pools in the lower extremities and this results in a reduced stroke volume. In addition, persons with tetraplegia will have a maximum heart rate of 110–130 beats·min^{-1}. Quadriplegic athletes performing a max test under (self-induced) AD conditions achieve a 10% faster race time performance than in normal condition. Norepinephrine levels (but not epinephrine) and maximum heart rate are significantly higher under AD conditions. Similar results in spinal cord injured athletes performing a wheelchair ergometer max test have been found. AD results in higher maximum heart rate (8%), maximum oxygen consumption (6%) and maximum power (7%). This shows that boosting can be a very potent performance enhancer, although some argue that AD is a normal physiologic response that enables athletes with high spinal lesions to use intrinsic capabilities of the body.

The IPC forbids athletes from competing in a dysreflexic state on health reasons. Although reports of severe complications after an AD event outside a clinical setting are rare, the severe hypertension puts the person at risk for cardiovascular complications. Before any IPC competition, athletes can be asked to take part in blood pressure measurements and refusal to do so may result in sanctions. If systolic blood pressure exceeds 180 mmHg, the subject will be tested for a second time after a 10 min rest period. If the second test again shows a blood pressure above 180 mmHg, the subject will be withdrawn from the competition. Spinal cord-injured athletes who have a lesion above T6 and are hypertensive should inform the relevant bodies via the usual TUE pathways. In addition, TUEs might be needed for medication commonly used by individuals with a spinal cord injury.

Fortunately, doping is not a big problem in adaptive rowing. However, sport scientific and medical support services for the adaptive rower should be aware of the possible conflict between anti-doping regulations and commonly prescribed medications in spinal cord injury or abnormal physiologic phenomena, such as autonomic dysreflexia.

References and recommended reading

Bernstein, I.A., Webber, O. & Woledge, R. (2002) An ergonomic comparison of rowing machine designs: possible implications for safety. *British Journal of Sports Medicine* **36**, 108–112.

Budgett, R. (1989) The road to success in international rowing. *British Journal of Sports Medicine* **23**, 49–50.

Budgett, R. & Fuller, G. (1989) Illness and injury in international rowing. *Clinics in Sports Medicine* **1**, 57–61.

Christiansen, E. & Kanstrup, I.L. (1997) Increased risk of stress fractures of the ribs in elite rowers. *Scandinavian Journal of Medicine and Science in Sports* **7**, 49–52.

Hickey, G.J., Fricker, P.A. & McDonald, W.A. (1997) Injuries to elite rowers over a 10 yr period. *Medicine and Science in Sports and Exercise* **29**, 1567–1572.

Holden, D. & Jackson, D.W. (1985) Stress fracture of the ribs in female rowers. *American Journal of Sports Medicine* **13**, 342–348.

International Paralympic Committee (2004) IPC Anti-doping code.

Karlson, K.A. (1998) Rib stress fractures in elite rowers: a case series and proposed mechanism. *American Journal of Sports Medicine* **26**, 516–519.

Koutedakis, Y., Frischknecht, R. & Murthy, M. (1997) Knee flexion to extension peak torque ratios and low-back injuries in highly active individuals. *International Journal of Sports Medicine* **18**, 290–295.

Manning, T.S., Plowman, S.A., Drake, G., *et al*. (2000) Intra-abdominal pressure and rowing: the effects of inspiring versus expiring during the drive. *Journal of Sports Medicine and Physical Fitness* **40**, 223–232.

McGregor, A., Anderton, L. & Gedroyc, W. (2002) The assessment of intersegmental motion and pelvic tilt in elite oarsmen. *Medicine and Science in Sports and Exercise* **34**, 1143–1149.

Morris, F.L., Smith, R.M., Payne, W.R., *et al*. (2000) Compressive and shear force generated in the lumbar spine of female rowers. *International Journal of Sports Medicine* **21**, 518–523.

O'Kane, J.W., Teitz, C.C. & Lind, B.K. (2003) Effect of pre-existing back pain on the incidence and severity of back pain in intercollegiate rowers. *American Journal of Sports Medicine* **31**, 80–82.

Redgrave, S. (1992) Injuries: prevention/cure. In: S. Redgrave, *Steven Redgrave's Complete Book of Rowing*. Partridge Press, London. pp. 200–217.

Roy, S.H., De Luca, C.J., Snyder-Mackler, L., Emley, M.S., Crenshaw, R.L. & Lyons, J.P. (1990) Fatigue, recovery and low back pain in varsity rowers. *Medicine and Science in Sports and Exercise* **22**, 463–469.

Rumball, J.S., Lebrun, C.M., Di Ciacca, S.R. & Orlando, K. (2005) Rowing injuries. *Sports Medicine* **35**, 537–555.

Schmid, A., Schmid-Trucksass, A., Huonker, M., *et al*. (2001) Catecholamine responses of high performance wheelchair athletes at rest and during exercise with autonomic dysreflexia. *International Journal of Sports Medicine* **22**, 2–7.

Stallard, M.C. (1980) Backache in oarsmen. *British Journal of Sports Medicine* **14**, 105–108.

Teitz, C.C. & O'Kane, J.W. Lind BK. (2003) Back pain in former intercollegiate rowers: a long-term follow-up study. *American Journal of Sports Medicine* **31**, 590–595.

Thomas, P.L. (1988) Thoracic back pain in rowers and butterfly swimmers: costovertebral subluxation. *British Journal of Sports Medicine* **22**, 81.

Volianitis, S., McConnell, A.K., Koutedakis, Y., McNaughton, L., Backx, K. & Jones, D.A. (2001) Inspiratory muscle training improves rowing performance. *Medicine and Science in Sports and Exercise* **33**, 803–809.

Warden, S.J., Gutschlag, F.R., Wajswelner, H. & Crossley, K.M. (2000) Aetiology of rib stress fractures in rowers. *Sports Medicine* **32**, 819–836.

Webborn, A.D. (1999) "Boosting" performance in disability sport. *British Journal of Sports Medicine* **33**, 74–75.

www.oara.org.uk

www.worldrowing.com

Chapter 12
Adaptive rowing

D. Hettinga

Introduction

Rowing competition for persons with physical, sensory and/or intellectual disability is a relative newcomer to the sport but has seen an exponential growth over the past years. Adaptive rowing has been included in the FISA World Championships since 2002 and will feature at the 2008 Beijing Para-lympic Games. Not only has the quality and quantity of the competition increased, but also the associated support functions, including scientific and medical services. These services are being confronted by questions that cannot be answered from able-bodied experience. This chapter describes such questions and suggests possible solutions.

Adaptive rowing includes arms only (A rowers; Fig. 12.1) and trunk-arms rowers (TA rowers). These rowers have impaired leg function and only use their arms and, to some extent, their trunk for rowing. A and TA rowers face a number of unique physiologic and musculoskeletal limitations in their training as in daily life. The training and exercise responses of other adaptive rowers, as those competing in the legs–trunk–arms class (LTA) (i.e., rowers with a visual, intellectual or minimal physical disability) are more similar to the responses of able-bodied rowers.

The spinal cord injured rower is taken as an example because this is the most common type of disability in the TA and A classifications. Moreover, spinal cord injury responds well to a new training technique described in this chapter. Functional

electrical stimulation assisted rowing (FES rowing) could alleviate the restrictions in the exercise response seen in rowers with a spinal cord injury.

Exercise response in rowers with spinal cord injury

Responses to exercise and training take place on two levels: peripherally (in the muscle) and centrally (in the heart, lungs and circulation). A lesion in the spinal cord can impact on both levels, although the impact depends on the location and the extent of the lesion. Complete lesions high in the spinal cord have a more pronounced effect on body functions than incomplete lesion lower in the spinal column. Classification in adaptive rowing is complex and includes medical and functional assessments, but a lesion at the 10th thoracic vertebra can be considered as the cut-off point between TA and A rowers. Moreover, most competitive rowers with a spinal cord injury have good hand function, which implies that their level of lesion in not above the first thoracic vertebra. Therefore, the majority of the spinal cord injured rowers competing in the A class have lesions in the thoracic spine, while TA rowers have lesions in the low thoracic or lumbar–sacral spine.

Peripheral limitations to exercise

The upper body muscular responses to exercise of TA and A rowers are similar to those of able-bodied rowers. Two differences can be identified:

141

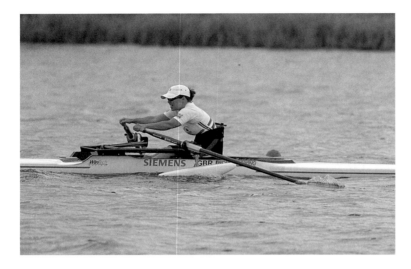

Fig. 12.1 Arms-only (A) rowing.

1 Diminished blood supply to the active muscle as a result of restriction in the central systems
2 Risk of musculoskeletal overuse in the upper body

The risk of overuse is a consequence of the fact that the spinal cord injured rower (and other wheelchair-bound athletes) has to perform all training and all other activities of daily life with solely his or her upper body. Consequently, the upper body (especially the shoulder joint) is taking more load than it is designed for. Up to 70% of long-term wheelchair users experience pain in the shoulder, arm or wrist, mostly as a result of shoulder impingement or carpal tunnel syndrome. The shoulder complaints most likely arise as a consequence of the high forces during weight transfers and/or the repetitive use of the shoulder during wheelchair propulsion. Wheelchair propulsion is a pushing action whereby the protractor muscles at the front of the shoulder are active, while the antagonist muscle at the rear of the shoulder and the back are only minimally active. This muscular imbalance is thought to have a major role in the etiology of overuse complaints in long-term wheelchair users.

Central limitations to exercise

The cardiovascular and respiratory responses to exercise are influenced by various factors, the most important being the amount of active muscle mass and the work rate of those muscles. This is where TA and A rowers are fundamentally different from LTA rowers and able-bodied rowers, because only the upper body is used for exercise. The largest muscles in the human body are located in the lower extremities and the inability to use these muscles during exercise results in lower total oxygen consumption ($\dot{V}O_2$) and lower exercise stimulus. Although highly trained Paralympic athletes can achieve high $\dot{V}O_2$ values with their upper body, it puts an excessive stress on a small muscle mass and this might have a role in the etiology of overuse syndrome.

More importantly, however, the inability to activate the large muscles in the lower extremities results in blood pooling in the legs. Muscular contractions are essential in pumping venous blood to the heart, especially in the legs where gravity forms a major challenge to venous return. Although the lower body of persons with spinal cord injury can adapt to some extent, it is likely that venous return is lower than normal. A reduced venous return leads to a lower preload and, subsequently, a lower stroke volume of the heart. Therefore, increases in cardiac output in exercising paraplegics is achieved by increases in heart rate and to a lesser degree by increases in stroke volume. Although maximum heart rate is, in most spinal cord injured rowers, close to normal, the limited stroke volume constrains maximum cardiac output but the horizontal position of the legs during rowing makes that problem less important.

These secondary consequences of a spinal cord injury are not only a limitation to training in (elite) athletes, but also result in an inability to exercise effectively and efficiently to prevent heart disease, diabetes and obesity.

In summary, the exercise response from a spinal cord injured rower is different from an able-bodied one in the following ways:
• The lower training stimulus to the heart, lungs and circulation because of the low maximal amount of active muscle mass
• The limitation in the stroke volume because of the absent muscle pump in the lower extremities
• The risk of overuse in the upper body because of the necessity to perform all training and all activities of daily life solely with the upper body

FES rowing

Functional electrical stimulation (FES) is a technique whereby small electrical currents from an external stimulator are sent through the skin to the muscle, which responds by contracting. This technique has been used extensively for lesions in the central nervous system that block the controlling signals from the brain to the muscles. The technology has been integrated with exercise systems such as cycling and rowing. The FES rowing machine consists of a standard Concept II ergometer that has been equipped with a back rest, strapping and leg stabilizers to provide the paraplegic rower with postural support. Electrodes on the skin over the quadriceps and hamstrings muscles are connected to a stimulator that is controlled by a switch on the handlebar of the ergometer. The drive phase is initiated by pushing the switch, which triggers quadriceps stimulation. Leg drive is followed by normal arm action after which the switch is released and the hamstrings are activated resulting in knee flexion. This allows persons with a spinal cord injury to activate their paralysed muscles and use a rowing machine more or less like the able rower. Besides the psychosocial benefits of being able to participate in a standard exercise, FES rowing could offer a

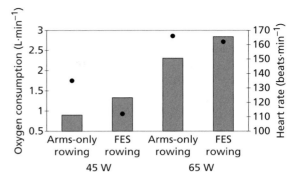

Fig. 12.2 Oxygen consumption (shaded columns) and heart rate (black dots) during FES rowing and arms-only rowing at similar power in a spinal cord injured subject (T5 complete lesion).

solution to secondary physiologic limitations and complications of spinal cord injury.

First of all, the problem around muscular imbalances in the shoulder of long-term wheelchair users can be prevented by using rowing as a shoulder retractor exercise. Electromyographic (EMG) studies show that the muscle activation pattern of the main muscles around the shoulder during rowing is similar to the pattern seen during shoulder retractor exercise. This could have an important role in re-establishing the balance between shoulder protractors and retractors.

Secondly, the electrical activation of the paralysed leg muscles re-activates the muscle pump and assists venous return. Figure 12.2 shows the heart rate and oxygen consumption of a spinal cord injured rower (complete lesion at T5) during arms-only and FES rowing. In both conditions, the subject was asked to row at a similar power. The results show that, at similar power, FES rowing resulted in consistently lower heart rate and higher oxygen consumption. In other words, the heart of the rower during FES rowing was able to deliver more oxygen to the muscles than during arms-only rowing. This implies a larger stroke volume during FES rowing, initiated by the active muscle pump in the lower extremities of the rower. Obviously the closer the rower gets to his or her physiologic maximum values, the smaller the differences, but oxygen consumption during FES rowing remains high. This results in a high training load on the central systems, while the

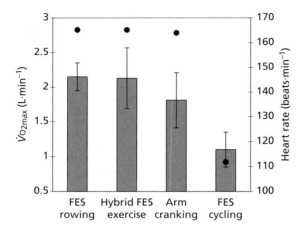

Fig. 12.3 Peak oxygen consumption ($\dot{V}_{O_{2max}}$, shaded columns) and peak heart rate (black dots) during FES rowing, hybrid FES exercise, arm cranking and FES cycling in five spinal cord injured subjects. Modified from Verellen *et al.* (2007).

training load for the peripheral systems is spread over a large muscle mass.

Figure 12.3 shows $\dot{V}_{O_{2max}}$ values in five subjects with spinal cord injury during four exercises. $\dot{V}_{O_{2max}}$ during FES rowing was higher than during FES cycling, and marginally higher than during arms cranking and a hybrid FES exercise (arms cranking combined with FES cycling). With the advantages of restoring muscular balances and the wide availability of rowing ergometers in mind, FES rowing would be the preferred option. Moreover, in a separate study, subjects reported that FES rowing at a certain power feels easier than arms-only rowing at similar or lower power.

Other benefits of FES training include muscle hypertrophy and improved blood circulation, which result in a decreased risk of pressure sores (decubitus). Pressure sores are relatively common in spinal cord injury and can be a significant medical complication with considerable discomfort and secondary disability for the individual. The increased muscle bulk after FES training acts as a natural cushion and the improved blood circulation gives better wound healing conditions.

The results of a series of studies suggest that FES rowing is a reliable high-intensity cardiovascular exercise that can have a role in the prevention of overuse syndrome, cardiovascular diseases, type 2 diabetes and obesity. Moreover, FES rowing is available at a competitive level. Since 2004, FES rowing is part of the British Indoor Rowing Championships and FES rowing also featured at the 2006 World Indoor Rowing Championships (CRASH-B). A few spinal cord injured rowers have used FES rowing in their training programs but larger studies need to confirm the value of FES rowing as a cross-training tool. The results suggest that FES rowing can be used as a high-intensity aerobic exercise that does not put individual muscles under excessive stress.

Recommended reading

http://www.fesrowing.org

Hettinga, D.M. (2006) The development and evaluation of functional electrical stimulation rowing for health, exercise and sport for persons with spinal cord injury. PhD thesis. Brunel University, London.

Olenik, L., Laskin, J.J., Burnham, R., Wheeler, G.D. & Steadward, R.D. (1995) Efficacy of rowing, backward wheeling and isolated scapular retractor exercise as remedial strength activities for wheelchair users: application of electromyography. *Paraplegia* **33**, 148–152.

Verellen, J., Vanlandewijck, Y., Andrews, B. & Wheeler, G.D. (2007) Cardiorespiratory responses during arm ergometry, functional electrial stimulation cycling and two hybrid exercise conditions in spinal cord injured. *Disability and Rehabilitation: Assistive Technologies* (in press).

Wheeler, G.D., Andrews, B., Lederer, R., *et al.* (2002) Functional electric stimulation-assisted rowing: Increasing cardiovascular fitness through functional electric stimulation rowing training in persons with spinal cord injury. *Archives of Physical Medicine and Rehabilitation* **83**, 1093–1099.

Chapter 13
Racing

S. Volianitis

Umpiring

At the start of an Olympic rowing race the boats are held by the stern on starting pontoons and the bows are aligned. The rower in the bow seat may raise his or her hand to indicate that the crew is not ready, up until the time when the starter conducts a roll call of the crews. At the start, the umpire is positioned centrally behind the boats on the start line. After the last crew has been named in the roll call by the aligner, the umpire checks that the aligner's flag is still raised and then says "Attention" and raises the red flag (Fig. 13.1).

After a clear pause, the umpire drops the red flag quickly to one side, simultaneously saying, "Go." Previously, the international rowing language was French and the starting command was, "Et vous prez, partez." For a quick start, instead of the roll call, the umpire says, "Quick start, attention" and then raises the red flag. In difficult wind conditions the umpire may decide to dispense with the normal and quick start procedures and revert to a rolling start, where the aligner directs the boats to proceed slowly down-course and maintain all boats in line abreast. At the earliest opportunity in the proximity of the start line when boats are in line, the aligner raises a white flag to indicate a line, after which the umpire starts the race by saying, "Rolling start, attention."

In the case of a false start, a bell is rung and the starter waves a red flag to recall the crews. Crews are allowed only one false start each before being eliminated. A restart can also be called for equipment breakage within 100 m of the start as marked by red buoys. Straying from a lane is punishable by the umpire by disqualification if interference takes place with another boat. Because the rowers face opposite from the direction of travel and the command "Port" means "Right" while "Starboard" means "Left", the directions of the umpire during the race are given to the crews both verbally and by using a white flag to avoid confusion (Fig. 13.2).

The winner is the boat whose bow touches the finish line first, monitored by the judges and a photo finish camera. The umpire must raise the white flag at the end of a race to signify that it has been completed in accordance with the rules and that there has been no protest.

Steering

The main factors that can affect the direction of the boat are the following:

1 *Weather conditions* The wind is the greatest force outside the boat that can change the boat's direction. Cross-wind is particularly challenging as the bow or the stern of the boat may be affected more. In the first case, the boat is pushed round with the wind and in the second the wind may push the stern round, forcing the boat to head into the wind.

2 *Balance of power* In selecting the crew, care must be taken to ensure an even distribution of power on

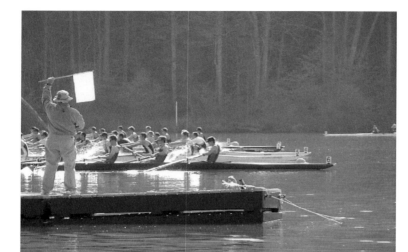

Fig. 13.1 The aligner at the start of a race.

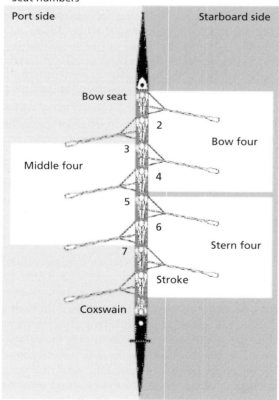

Fig. 13.2 Terminology and seating arrangement of an eight.

each side of the boat. In deciding crew positions, the leverage advantage of the bowman should be accounted for. The problem of leverage is to some extent overcome by the rigging of bow and stroke on the same side with two and three together in the middle of the boat.

Steering is performed by adjusting the pressure on the oars in sculling boats (1× and 2×) or by a rudder used either by a coxswain (2+, 4+, 8+) or a steersman (2–, 4–, 4×), who is one of the rowers. A boat can be steered only if it has speed in relation to the surrounding water. If the boat is traveling at the same speed as the surrounding water, the rudder's deflection will not change the boat's direction and this is an important consideration in rowing races held in the same direction as the flow of the river. Having the rudder at the stern places the action lines of the forces applied distant to the boat's center of gravity and produces rotary motion by utilizing the law of leverage (Fig. 13.3).

Effective rudder pressure depends on the traveling speed, the rudder angle, the lever arm (consisting of the distance from the center of gravity of the immersed part of the boat, the so-called center of lateral resistance, to the rudder). The most effective steering effect occurs at an angle of 30–35° to the neutral position. The ensuing torque produces rotation of the boat around its center of gravity. The

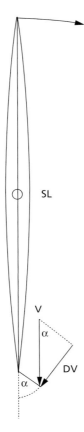

Fig. 13.3 Effect of pressure on the stern rudder. α, rudder angle; DV, rudder pressure; SL, center of gravity of the immersed body of the boat; V, boat speed.

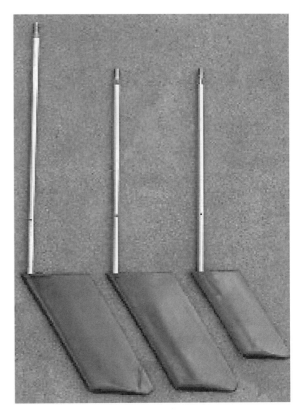

Fig. 13.4 Rudders.

radii of the turning arcs at bow and stern vary in size depending on the position of the center of gravity. It is important to understand that the boat does not change its course immediately after the rudder is applied but continues on its path although pointing in a new direction. The boat, in fact, skids for a period and at this time much resistance builds up along the complete side of the hull. In effect, the width of the boat is temporarily increased. As the effectiveness of steering depends on the speed of the boat, the rudders designed for slow or fast boats are long and flat or short and high (deep), respectively. Application of the rudder involves hydrodynamic pressure and suction, which further increase the already existing turbulence of the water, and

increases the skin resistance. These side effects can be avoided by streamlining the rudder, in relation to the body of the boat. Steering is improved when the rudder is moved completely out of range of the wake and fitted under the keel in relatively undisturbed water (fin rudder). The desired effect is obtained even with relatively small rudders, because the entire rudder surface is overflowed fully by the water. Modern boats are fitted with interchangeable rudder blades to enable the steering to be adjusted to meet the prevailing conditions (wind, wave formation; Fig. 13.4). Another useful way to improve steering is by fitting a fin rudder near the stern. The rudder that is fixed to the stern of the boat affects the steering in a different way from a rudder positioned some distance from the stern post (or closer to the fin). A rudder at the stern helps to hold the boat on course but is more ponderous in its steering. A rudder fitted nearer to the fin is more sensitive and is inclined to allow the boat to skid more than a conventional rudder.

If the rudder has produced a change in the boat's direction, the boat continues to turn further in that direction even after the rudder has been returned to the neutral position. Therefore, the rudder should be returned to the neutral position before the bow of the boat aims at the desired location.

The coxswain

The word coxswain is derived from the Saxon, *cockes* ("for, or of the boat") and *swain* from the old Norse word *Sveinn* ("servant"); thus, "servant of the boat." The main duties of the coxswain during a race, besides steering, are to provide rhythm, encouragement and race information to the rowers (Figs 13.5 & 13.6).

Steering can be difficult as rowing boats are designed for speed, not maneuverability. There are two schools of thought on steering. Many coxswains advocate that the rudder should only be applied when the blades are in the water (the drive phase) while others insist that the rudder can be applied at any time, but only slightly. The argument stems from the fact that changing the hydrodynamics of the shell by steering upsets the balance of the boat. The boat is most stable when the blades are in the water and least stable on the recovery. It is advantageous to the speed of the shell if it is balanced throughout the whole stroke.

Steering tips

Handling and steering of the boat varies depending on whether the body of water is still, as in all Fédération Internationale des Sociétés d'Aviron (FISA) courses, or there is a current, as in most head races held on rivers. In any case, because every deflection of the rudder means loss in speed, steering should be minimal. On still water, approaching a dock perpendicular to the bank must be from a direction that the wind, if any, drives the boat to the dock, while when pushing-off the dock should be from the side where the wind drives the boat away from the dock. On fast flowing water, docking and pushing away from the dock (parallel to the bank) must be against the current. During docking, the approach should be at an acute angle and then the boat should turn parallel to the dock. The rudder should be firmly held at the neutral position when rowing backwards.

Small waves can be crossed at right angles, while for long or larger waves the boat should be parallel

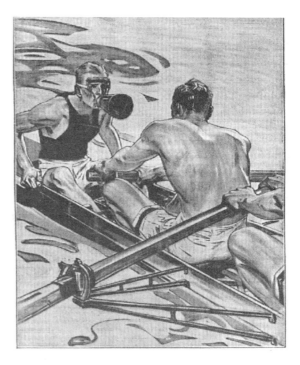

Fig. 13.6 The coxswain.

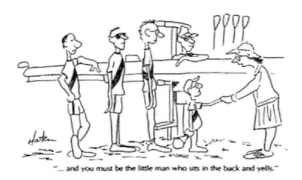

"... and you must be the little man who sits in the back and yells."

Fig. 13.5 The coxswain.

to the wave and the rudder secured in neutral position with blades flat on the water. Abrupt movements during steering should be avoided as they can disturb the balance of the boat. In side winds, the coxswain can help the balance of the boat by sitting somewhat towards the side of the wind.

International rowing courses with six-lane racing give no leeway and the crews merely keep to their own lanes. In head races, however, the positioning of the boat, even by a few feet, where the stream is faster, or a wind, or where the banks are uneven, can provide a significant advantage. River flow is driven by the hydrostatic pressure gradient, which is constant across the cross-section of the river. This would mean that the stream flows at an equal speed at all points within the cross-section, because each point is driven by the same force. However, because of the viscosity of the water, the flow is slower near the fixed boundaries (riverbed and banks) and faster near the free boundary (surface, because the air offers relatively little resistance to flow), and the quickest flow is furthest from the fixed boundary, which means away from the sides and where the river is deepest. As in most rivers the width is larger than the depth, the flow rate is mostly determined by the depth rather than the distance from the sides. The stream flows in a straight line and change course only when deflected by the riverbanks or obstacles in the water. The stream does not therefore naturally follow the curves in the riverbed but crosses from side to side as directed by the banks. Where the river is wide and straight, the main stream concentrates in the middle, or where the water is deeper, but when a bend in the river occurs the force of the stream is carried towards the outside bank of the bend. When there is floodwater and the strength of the stream consequently increases, often some of the stream is pushed in the opposite direction under the shelter of the bend. This is the main reason for not taking the shortest distance round a bend when the stream is flowing fast.

When racing with a fast stream, the boats should keep to the inside of the middle going into the bend and to the outside of the middle coming out of the bend. When racing against the stream, boats should approach on the inside of the bend as close to the

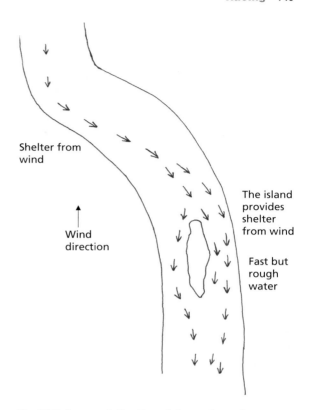

Fig. 13.7 Force and direction of stream shown by arrows

bank as possible and the coxswain/steersman should always seek shelter from the stream; this may be a bend in the river, a bay, an obstacle offering shelter, a bridge buttress or an island. Where the river runs wide the stream slows down but where it narrows the stream may be fierce, especially in the winter months. If there is no stream at all, the shortest possible route is preferred.

When crossing the stream or when taking a corner, a fast stream may push against the bow first and then the stern. Care must be taken when approaching a river corner because the stream will affect the bow first as soon as the corner is reached (Fig. 13.7).

The wind is one of the most important factors in boat racing, not only for its effect on the speed of the boat, but also for its effect on the crew members. When the wind blows against the stream the water gets rough—the harder the wind blows and the faster the stream, the rougher it becomes. The water is roughest where the wind, or stream, is greatest and the coxswain/steersman has to choose either the rough water, where there is fast stream and head wind, or the calm water with no stream and little wind.

The height of the riverbanks is also important. High, or walled, banks may provide shelter from the wind but at the same time the water may be rough, as the waves do not have a chance to subside. River-banks that rise gradually provide a damper for waves and rough water, and the water is calmer.

Recommended reading

www.worldrowing.com

Herberger, E., *et al.* (1983) *Rudern* (*Rowing*): *The GDR text of oarsmanship*. Sports Books Publisher.

Appendix
Development of performance

Niels H. Secher and T. Vogelsang

For the competitive oarsman, results obtained in an international regatta and, notably, in the Fédération Internationale des Sociétés d'Aviron (FISA) regatta of the year, represent the state of the art. Many sports disciplines are described by national, world and Olympic records, but for rowing, such defined performance characteristics can not be provided. The obvious reason is that for any given regatta, the recorded race time is influenced not only by the ability of the crew to row but also by the weather conditions. A head wind results in a much slower speed relative to the shore than a tailwind, and a side wind also challenges the balance of the boat to make the race slower than would be the case under neutral weather conditions.

Despite the various wind circumstances under which a regatta is held, it is clear that results in rowing improve with the passage of time. This can be seen when the results are compared for the same race that has been held over many years, for example, the men's eight event at the Royal Henley Regatta (Fig. 1.6). The improvement is also visible in the results of the FISA regatta held on a new venue each year as presented in the tables and figures of this appendix. With the marked influence of wind on the results, the improvement of rowing results is illustrated most clearly for those events that have been represented in every regatta since the first European championship in 1893 (single scull, coxed four, and the eight; Tables A.1, 4, and 8). Conversely, the increase in the distance for women from 1000 to 2000 m, and the late introduction of some of the lightweight events, makes the

database comparatively small and the calculated regression lines are dominated by the prevalent weather conditions.

Considering that the prevailing weather changes at random, the regression line for each rowing event represents the time a typical race would be expected to last. Furthermore, the intercept of the regression line for 2007 may be taken to represent the expected time for the race in the upcoming FISA regatta under the premise that weather does not dominate the result. Therefore, the calculated time for 2007 may be compared to the World records on a rowing ergometer (Table 1.3). This is the case not only for the single scull, but also for pairs, fours and the eight with the introduction of ergometers connected to each other and working together on slides.

The basis for the plot of results obtained in the FISA regatta presented in the figures of this chapter is that they represent the same lengths of the course. Thus, the 3000 m race of the first European championship is not taken into consideration. Also, as indicated in the tables, those results obtained on rivers with an assumed significant current, have been disregarded in the calculations of the regression lines. Yet, there remains hidden bias. For the first 75 years (approximately) of the FISA regatta, the course was defined as 2000 m. That meant that the long eight-oared boat had to row the shortest distance. With the 2000 m now measured from the stern at the starting line to the finish line, the "true" improvement of the results is some 3 s more impressive than indicated by the figures.

Overall, the improvement of the results is by about one second per year (Table 1.5) and many factors can be considered to contribute to that improvement. When looking at the boats used for the early FISA regattas, they appear remarkably similar to those used today. Yet, it is not difficult to see differences in all parts of the construction. The riggers are now much more stable, the distance travelled by the seat is longer and often "going through the pin" and, accordingly, the style of rowing has changed to include more power with the legs and less "swing" of the body. Not only does the modern rowing style allow for the development of greater power, but it also decreases the up and down movement of the body's center of gravity and, thereby, makes the boat move more smoothly through the water. In the pairs and fours, the coxswain has been moved to the front of the boat and he now lies down rather than sits up, again making the movement of the boat more stable. Further improvement is in the shape of the oar (Fig. 1.16). The blade of the early oar and sculls was very narrow indeed and the shape has changed to become more rounded as exemplified by the Macon type blade that, in turn, has been replaced by the now dominant "big blade". Obviously, the boat has changed from being made of wood to a plastic or carbon fibre construction and, similarly, the oars are of carbon fibre rather than of wood. Accordingly, it is now possible to standardize the boats and the current weight limits for the boats are presented in Table 1.2. Also, the boats are standardized in the sense that the sliding rigger system (Fig. 1.15) winning the World single scull championship for Peter Kolbe in 1981 and 1982 (Table A.4) is no longer permitted.

As mentioned, early regattas took place on very different venues and at one time over a different distance but, gradually, the rowing course has become a dedicated stadium. The first such rowing stadium was the Bosbaan in Amsterdam constructed for the Olympic Games in 1928. Similarly, the Xochimilco venue in Mexico City, the course in Munich, and many more courses have been constructed for their respective Olympic games. But standardization of the race course goes beyond the construction of the course, including ~30° banks in order to attenuate a rebound of waves created not only by the wind but also by the racing boats, themselves,

and, more significantly, by the motor boats used by the umpires and the rescue team following each race. Also, the buoy system separating each lane has been standardized so as to make it difficult for the blade of the oar to get caught up as was the case for the "hard luck" Danish coxless four during the finals of the European championships at the Bosbaan 1964.

With all these technical improvements, the figures of this chapter, including the 95% confidence interval for the regression lines (dots), illustrate that there is much more stability in the results of the FISA regatta than was the case in the early years. It may be speculated whether the technical changes give room to detect a contribution by the oarsmen to the ever improving results obtained. There is every reason to believe that a substantial part of the improvement of results are strongly related to an enhanced selection and training of the rowers. Results improve with the size of the oarsmen and, in general, due to enhanced nutrition, the height of the population has increased by one centimetre per decade, at least until recently. So, even among a non-selected group of young people, therefore, the team might be expected to become gradually larger over the 100 years or more that the FISA regatta has taken place. Considering that the rowing team has always been made up of rather large individuals (Chapter 3), it has become easier to find extremely tall and muscular rowers. The size of the winning teams has definitely increased over the years. For the women's events, there has been a reduced emphasis on the selection of large individuals. For the 1000 m race, the influence of body mass on the result is even more significant than for the current 2000 m race. Thus it may be that the progression of the height and weight of women rowers winning international championships has declined somewhat.

The possibility to train has also improved considerably as society in many countries has become richer. In the early years, rowing was dominated by people who had to work or study and rowing, even on an international level, was a leisure time pursuit. This is in contrast to the more or less professional life that many international oarsmen now live and the national team is surrounded by educated coaches together with physiologists, physiotherapists, medical doctors, and professional managers. It would be meaningless to arrange a professional championship as was established early in the 19th century (Fig. 1.14), or the FISA regatta may be considered to represent a professional championship. Accordingly, the FISA championship is now won by teams in their late twenties while, previously, it was an exception to find a competitive oarsman older that 30 years of age and "Nations Cup" for rowers under 23 years may be considered the present regatta that simulates the amateur championship. Yet, even these young rowers may come out of schools where competitive rowing is part of the program.

Not only is much more time spent rowing than just a generation ago, but bad weather conditions are compensated for by training camps over long periods under favorable weather conditions. Furthermore, outside such training camps, the widespread use of rowing ergometers allows for year-round rowing to an extent that was not possible with the use of indoor rowing tanks (Fig. 1.18).

With much more time spent rowing and comparatively less time spent on, e.g. gymnastics, weightlifting, circuit training, and running different distances, the technique of rowing has improved. This is reflected in a lower oxygen uptake at a given rowing speed for teams training over long distances compared to those training at a high intensity over a relatively short distance. This was inspired, at least to some extent, by the German coach Karl Adam (Fig. 1.20).

It may be considered that, with the standardization of the rowing course and the weight of the boats and, furthermore, with the stability of the size of the population in many countries, further improvements in rowing results will depend on the individual rower. Accordingly, the result from the eight event at the Royal Henley regatta indicates that further improvement of results will be slow (Fig. 1.6). With internationally competitive rowing representing something similar to a normal job, there is a limit to how much more can be gained by training. Improved results will depend on enhanced quality of training and/or the appearance of rowers with extraordinary talent. Such talent identification is facilitated by the sport of rowing, starting with the five nations forming FISA in 1892 (p. 17), gradually covering the whole world. An increased interest in rowing among children may be important both to identify the talented rower and to learn superb technique.

Recommended reading

Secher, N.H. (1973) Development of results in international rowing championships 1983–1971. *Medicine and Scence in Sports and Exercise* **5**, 195–199.
Secher, N.H. & Vaage, O. (1983) Rowing performance, a mathematical model based on body dimensions as exemplified by body weight. *European Journal of Applied Physiology* **52**, 88–93.

Table A.1 Winning results in men's single scull (M1x).

Year	Event	Place	Winner	Time (min s)	Comment	Year	Event	Place	Winner	Time (min s)	Comment
1893	EC	Orta	BEL		3000 m	1903	EC	Venice	FRA	8 40	
1894	EC	Macon	FRA	7 15		1904	EC	Paris	SUI		
1895	EC	Ostende	BEL	8 10		1904	OG	St Louis	USA	10 08	River
1896	EC	Geneva	SUI			1905	EC	Ghent	ALS	7 51	
1897	RC	Pallanza	BEL	8 55		1906	EC	Pallanza	FRA	8 35	
1898	EC	Torin	BEL	7 30		1906	OG	Athens	FRA	5 53.4	1000 m
1899	EC	Ostende	FRA	8 08		1907	EC	Strasbourg	FRA	8 24	
1900	EC	Paris	FRA	6 09	1700 m	1908	EC	Lucerne	FRA	5 52	River
1900	OG	Paris	FRA	7 35.6	River	1908	OG	Henley	GBR	9 26.0	2414 m
1901	EC	Zürich	FRA	9 56	River	1909	EC	Juvisy	ITA	7 43	
1902	EC	Strasbourg	ITA	8 51.4		1910	EC	Ostend	FRA	7 55	

(Continued.)

Table A.1 *Continued.*

Year	Event	Place	Winner	Time (min s)	Comment	Year	Event	Place	Winner	Time (min s)	Comment
1911	EC	Como	ITA	8 14		1964	EC	Amsterdam	URS	7 05.19	
1912	EC	Geneva	BEL	8 47.0		1964	OG	Tokyo	URS	8 22.51	
1912	OG	Stockholm	GBR	7 47.6		1965	EC	Duisburg	GER	7 42.10	
1913	EC	Ghent	GER			1966	WC	Bled	USA	7 05.92	
1920	EC	Macon	SUI	7 35		1967	EC	Vichy	RDA	7 59.88	
1920	OG	Antwerp	USA	7 35.0		1967	NAC	St Catharines	DEN	7 41.40	
1921	EC	Amsterdam	NDL	7 16.4	1800 m	1968	OG	Mexico	NDL	7 47.80	
1922	EC	Barcelona	SUI	9 06		1969	EC	Klagenfurt	ARG	7 45.79	
1923	EC	Como	SUI	8 02.6		1970	WC	St Catharines	ARG	7 16.54	
1924	EC	Zürich	SUI	8 20		1971	EC	Copenhagen	ARG	6 57.99	
1924	OG	Paris	GBR	7 49.2		1972	OG	Munich	URS	7 10.12	
1925	EC	Prague	NDL	6 40.2	River	1973	EC	Moscow	RFA	8 02.77	
1926	EC	Lucerne	NDL	7 44.4		1974	WC	Lucerne	RDA	7 20.11	
1927	EC	Como	ITA	7 50.0		1975	WC	Nottingham	RFA	7 10.08	
1928	OG	Amsterdam	AUS	7 11.0		1976	OG	Montreal	FIN	7 29.03	
1929	EC	Bydgoszcz	NDL	6 32.8	1750 m	1977	WC	Amsterdam	RDA	7 12.22	
1930	EC	Liege	HON	6 26.6	River	1978	WC	L. Karapiro	RFA	7 06.01	
1931	EC	Paris	SUR	7 06		1979	WC	Bled	FIN	6 58.27	
1932	EC	Belgrad	ITA	7 18.2		1980	OG	Moscow	FIN	7 09.61	
1932	OG	Los Angeles	AUS	7 44.4		1981	WC	Munich	RFA	7 45.32	Fig.1.15
1933	EC	Budapest	POG	6 28.4	2300 m	1982	WC	Lucerne	RDA	7 00.67	Fig.1.15
1934	EC	Lucerne	GER	7 38.2		1983	WC	Duisburg	RFA	6 49.88	
1935	EC	Berlin	POG	7 54		1984	OG	Los Angeles	FIN	7 00.24	
1936	OG	Berlin	GER	8 21.5		1985	WC	Hazewinkel	FIN	6 48.08	
1937	EC	Amsterdam	SUI	7 14.4		1986	WC	Nottingham	RFA	6 54.90	
1938	EC	Milano	GER	7 40.1		1987	WC	Copenhagen	RDA	7 37.48	
1947	EC	Lucerne	FRA	7 23.4		1988	OG	Seoul	RDA	6 49.86	
1948	OG	Henley	AUS	7 24.4	River	1990	WC	Tasmania	RUS	7 22.15	
1949	EC	Amsterdam	USA	7 30.8		1991	WC	Vienna	GER	6 41.29	
1950	EC	Milano	DEN	7 25.7		1992	OG	Barcelona	GER	6 51.40	
1951	EC	Macon	DEN	7 32.1		1993	WC	Racice	CAN	6 59.03	
1952	OG	Helsingfors	URS	8 12.8		1994	WC	Indianapolis	GER	6 46.33	
1953	EC	Copenhagen	YOU	7 14.6		1995	WC	Tampere	SLO	6 52.93	
1954	EC	Amsterdam	SUI	7 12.4		1996	OG	Atlanta	SUI	6 44.85	
1955	EC	Ghent	POG	7 08.3		1997	WC	Aiguebelette	USA	6 44.86	
1956	EC	Bled	URS	7 24.5		1998	WC	Cologne	NZL	6 39.65	
1956	OG	Melbourne	URS	8 02.5		1999	WC	St Catharines	NZL	6 36.68	
1957	EC	Duisburg	AUS	7 02.9		2000	OG	Sydney	NZL	6 48.90	
1958	EC	Poznan	AUS	7 33.6		2001	WC	Lucerne	NOR	6 43.04	
1959	EC	Macon	URS	6 58.9		2002	WC	Seville	GER	6 36.33	
1960	OG	Rome	URS	7 13.96		2003	WC	Milano	NOR	6 46.15	
1961	EC	Prague	URS	7 21.61		2004	OG	Athens	NOR	6 49.30	
1962	WC	Lucerne	URS	7 07.09		2005	WC	Gifu	NZL	7 16.42	
1963	EC	Copenhagen	TCH	7 11.84		2006	WC	Eton	NZL	6 35.40	

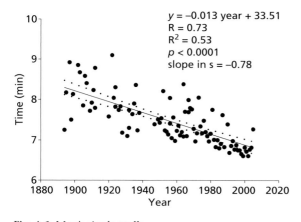

Fig. A.1 Men's single sculls.

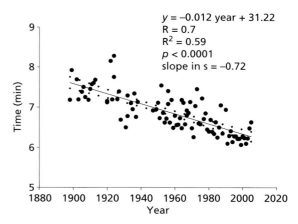

Fig. A.2 Men's double sculls.

Table A.2 Winning results in men's double sculls (M2x).

Year	Event	Place	Winner	Time (min s)	Comment	Year	Event	Place	Winner	Time (min s)	Comment
1898	EC	Torin	FRA	7 11		1926	EC	Lucerne	SUI	7 11.8	
1899	EC	Ostende	BEL	7 55		1927	EC	Como	SUI	7 23.2	
1900	EC	Paris	FRA	6 13.2	1700 m	1928	OG	Amsterdam	USA	6 41.4	
1901	EC	Zürich	FRA	9 39	River	1929	EC	Bydgoszcz	SUI	6 11.8	1750 m
1902	EC	Strasbourg	BEL	7 41.6		1930	EC	Liege	SUI	6 07	River
1903	EC	Venice	BEL	7 11.2		1931	EC	Paris	SUI	6 30	
1904	EC	Paris	FRA			1932	EC	Belgrad	HON	6 47	
1904	OG	St Louis	USA	10 03.2	River	1932	OG	Los Angeles	USA	7 17.4	
1905	EC	Ghent	BEL	7 23		1933	EC	Budapest	FRA	6 20.6	2300 m
1906	EC	Pallanza	BEL	7 30		1934	EC	Lucerne	SUI	7 06	
1907	EC	Strasbourg	ITA	7 15		1935	EC	Berlin	POG	6 56.7	
1908	EC	Lucerne	BEL	7 57.6	River	1936	OG	Berlin	GBR	7 20.8	
1909	EC	Juvisy	BEL	7 11		1937	EC	Amsterdam	GER	6 45.3	
1910	EC	Ostende	FRA	7 27		1938	EC	Milano	ITA	7 07.5	
1911	EC	Como	ITA	7 34		1947	EC	Lucerne	NDL	6 55.4	
1912	EC	Geneva	ITA	7 36		1948	OG	Henley	GBR	6 51.3	River
1913	EC	Ghent	FRA	7 41		1949	EC	Amsterdam	DEN	6 57.2	
1920	EC	Macon	FRA	7 07.4		1950	EC	Milano	DEN	7 06.5	
1920	OG	Antwerp	USA	7 09.0		1951	EC	Macon	SUI	6 44	
1921	EC	Amsterdam	NDL	5 49.00	1800 m	1952	OG	Helsingfors	ARG	7 32.2	
1922	EC	Barcelona	SUI	8 09.00		1953	EC	Copenhagen	SUI	6 51.4	
1923	EC	Como	SUI	7 11.6		1954	EC	Amsterdam	GER	6 37.2	
1924	EC	Zürich	SUI	8 17.00		1955	EC	Ghent	POG	6 43.1	
1924	OG	Paris	USA	7 45		1956	EC	Bled	URS	7 05.0	
1925	EC	Prague	SUI	6 10.2	River	1956	OG	Melbourne	URS	7 24.0	

(*Continued.*)

Table A.2 *Continued.*

Year	Event	Place	Winner	Time (min s)	Comment	Year	Event	Place	Winner	Time (min s)	Comment
1957	EC	Duisburg	URS	6 37.0		1981	WC	Munich	RDA	6 41.99	
1958	EC	Poznan	URS	7 10.7		1982	WC	Lucerne	NOR	6 23.66	
1959	EC	Macon	URS	6 29.49		1983	WC	Duisburg	RDA	6 20.17	
1960	OG	Rome	TCH	6 47.50		1984	OG	Los Angeles	USA	6 37.87	
1961	EC	Prague	URS	6 33.61		1985	WC	Hazewinkel	RDA	6 15.49	
1962	WC	Lucerne	FRA	6 33.90		1986	WC	Nottingham	ITA	6 30.33	
1963	EC	Copenhagen	TCH	6 43.54		1987	WC	Copenhagen	BUL	7 03.33	
1964	EC	Amsterdam	URS	6 28.90		1988	OG	Seoul	NDL	6 21.13	
1964	OG	Tokyo	URS	7 10.66		1990	WC	Tasmania	AUT	6 56.37	
1965	EC	Duisburg	SUI	7 06.42		1991	WC	Vienna	NDL	6 06.14	
1966	WC	Bled	SUI	6 34.89		1992	OG	Barcelona	AUS	6 17.32	
1967	EC	Vichy	SUI	6 47.85		1993	WC	Racice	FRA	6 24.69	
1967	NAC	St Catharines	SUI	6 55.35		1994	WC	Indianapolis	NOR	6 08.33	
1968	OG	Mexico	URS	6 51.82		1995	WC	Tampere	DEN	6 17.01	
1969	EC	Klagenfurt	USA	7 07.82		1996	OG	Atlanta	ITA	6 16.98	
1970	WC	St Catharines	DEN	6 28.68		1997	WC	Aiguebelette	GER	6 13.35	
1971	EC	Copenhagen	RDA	6 15.27		1998	WC	Cologne	GER	6 13.20	
1972	OG	Munich	URS	7 01.77		1999	WC	St Catharines	SLO	6 04.37	
1973	WC	Moscow	RDA	7 26.95		2000	OG	Sydney	SLO	6 16.63	
1974	WC	Lucerne	RDA	6 35.95		2001	WC	Lucerne	HUN	6 14.16	
1975	WC	Nottingham	NOR	6 31.49		2002	WC	Seville	HUN	6 05.74	
1976	OG	Montreal	NOR	7 13.20		2003	WC	Milano	FRA	6 13.93	
1977	WC	Amsterdam	GBR	6 42.83		2004	OG	Athens	FRA	6 29.00	
1978	WC	L. Karapiro	NOR	6 51.23		2005	WC	Gifu	SLO	6 37.61	
1979	WC	Bled	NOR	6 26.98		2006	WC	Eton	FRA	6 07.60	
1980	OG	Moscow	RDA	6 24.33							

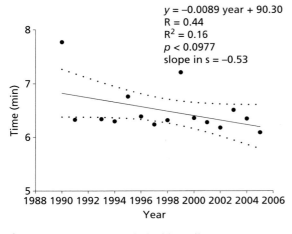

$y = -0.0089\ \text{year} + 90.30$
$R = 0.44$
$R^2 = 0.16$
$p < 0.0977$
slope in s $= -0.53$

Fig. A.3 Lightweight men's double sculls.

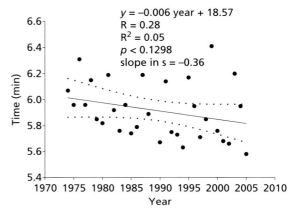

$y = -0.006\ \text{year} + 18.57$
$R = 0.28$
$R^2 = 0.05$
$p < 0.1298$
slope in s $= -0.36$

Fig. A.4 Men's quadruple sculls.

Table A.3 Winning results in lightweight double scull (LM2x).

Year	Event	Place	Winner	Time	Year	Event	Place	Winner	Time
1990	WC	Tasmania	USA	7 46.15	1999	WC	St Catharines	ITA	7 12.46
1991	WC	Vienna	GER	6 20.04	2000	OG	Sydney	POL	6 21.75
1993	WC	Racice	AUS	6 20.64	2001	WC	Lucerne	ITA	6 16.75
1994	WC	Indianapolis	ITA	6 18.10	2002	WC	Seville	ITA	6 10.80
1995	WC	Tampere	ITA	6 45.56	2003	WC	Milano	ITA	6 30.60
1996	OG	Atlanta	ITA	6 23.47	2004	OG	Athens	POL	6 20.93
1997	WC	Aiguebelette	POL	6 14.57	2005	WC	Gifu	HUN	6 05.10
1998	WC	Cologne	POL	6 19.11	2006	WC	Eton	DEN	6 11.42

Table A.4 Winning results in men's quadruple sculls (M4x).

Year	Event	Place	Winner	Time (min s)	Year	Event	Place	Winner	Time (min s)
1974	WC	Lucerne	RDA	6 04.01	1991	WC	Vienna	RUS	6 08.39
1975	WC	Nottingham	RDA	5 57.44	1992	OG	Barcelona	GER	5 45.17
1976	OG	Montreal	RDA	6 18.65	1993	WC	Racice	GER	5 43.99
1977	WC	Amsterdam	RDA	5 57.44	1994	WC	Indianapolis	ITA	5 37.68
1978	WC	L. Karapiro	RDA	6 08.94	1995	WC	Tampere	ITA	6 10.09
1979	WC	Bled	RDA	5 50.70	1996	OG	Atlanta	GER	5 56.93
1980	OG	Moscow	RDA	5 49.81	1997	WC	Aiguebelette	ITA	5 42.50
1981	WC	Munich	RDA	6 11.37	1998	WC	Cologne	ITA	5 51.19
1982	WC	Lucerne	RDA	5 55.50	1999	WC	St Catharines	GER	6 24.37
1983	WC	Duisburg	RFA	5 45.97	2000	OG	Sydney	ITA	5 45.56
1984	OG	Los Angeles	RFA	5 57.55	2001	WC	Lucerne	GER	5 40.89
1985	WC	Hazewinkel	CAN	5 44.57	2002	WC	Seville	GER	5 39.57
1986	WC	Nottingham	URS	5 47.41	2003	WC	Milano	GER	6 12.26
1987	WC	Copenhagen	URS	6 11.25	2004	OG	Athens	RUS	5 56.85
1988	OG	Seoul	ITA	5 53.37	2005	WC	Gifu	POL	5 34.96
1990	WC	Tasmania	RUS	5 40.44	2006	WC	Eton	POL	5 38.99

Table A.5 Winning results in men's coxless pair (M2–).

Year	Event	Place	Winner	Time (min s)	Comment	Year	Event	Place	Winner	Time (min s)	Comment
1900	OG	Paris	BEL	7 49.4	River	1926	EC	Lucerne	SUI	7 44.6	
1904	OG	St Louis	USA			1927	EC	Como	ITA	7 54.6	
1908	OG	Henley	GBR	9 41.0	2414 m	1928	OG	Amsterdam	GER	7 06.4	
1920	OG	Antwerp	ITA	7 56		1929	EC	Bydgoszcz	ITA	6 40.2	1750 m
1924	EC	Zürich	SUI	7 41		1930	EC	Liege	POL	6 02	River
1924	OG	Paris	NDL	8 19.4		1931	EC	Paris	NDL	7 01.6	
1925	EC	Prague	SUI	6 42	River	1932	EC	Relgrad	SUI	7 14.2	

(*Continued.*)

Table A.5 *Continued.*

Year	Event	Place	Winner	Time (min s)	Comment	Year	Event	Place	Winner	Time (min s)	Comment
1932	OG	Los Angeles	GBR	8 00.0		1972	OG	Munich	RDA	6 53.16	
1933	EC	Budapest	HON	6 24	2300 m	1973	EC	Moscow	ROU	7 39.10	
1934	EC	Lucerne	AUS	7 47.6		1974	WC	Lucerne	RDA	6 59.09	
1935	EC	Berlin	HON	7 55.4		1975	WC	Nottingham	RDA	7 06.40	
1936	OG	Berlin	GER	8 16.1		1976	OG	Montreal	RDA	7 23.31	
1937	EC	Amsterdam	ITA	7 18.5		1977	WC	Amsterdam	URS	7 06.19	
1938	EC	Milano	GER	7 23.2		1978	WC	L. Karapiro	RDA	7 00.92	
1947	EC	Lucerne	DEN	7 21.1		1979	WC	Bled	RDA	6 42.63	
1948	OG	Henley	GBR	7 21.1	River	1980	OG	Moscow	RDA	6 48.01	
1949	EC	Amsterdam	SUI	7 28.2		1981	WC	Munich	URS	7 15.06	
1950	EC	Milano	SUI	7 17.5		1982	WC	Lucerne	NOR	6 41.98	
1951	EC	Macon	BEL	7 32.2		1983	WC	Duisburg	RDA	6 35.85	
1952	OG	Helsingfors	USA	8 20.7		1984	OG	Los Angeles	ROU	6 45.39	
1953	EC	Copenhagen	URS	7 03.1		1985	WC	Hazewinkel	URS	6 38.39	
1954	RC	Amsterdam	DEN	6 59.2		1986	WC	Nottingham	URS	6 42.37	
1955	EC	Ghent	HON	6 59.1		1987	WC	Copenhagen	GBR	7 11.20	
1956	EC	Bled	URS	7 10.5		1988	OG	Seoul	GBR	6 36.84	
1956	OG	Melbourne	USA	7 55.4		1990	WC	Tasmania	GER	7 07.91	
1957	EC	Duisburg	GBR	6 57.0		1991	WC	Vienna	GBR	6 21.35	
1958	EC	Poznan	FIN	7 52.4		1992	OG	Barcelona	GBR	6 27.72	
1959	EC	Macon	GER	6 44.7		1993	WC	Racice	GBR	6 36.98	
1960	OG	Rome	URS	7 02.1		1994	WC	Indianapolis	GBR	6 18.65	
1961	EC	Prague	GER	7 01.9		1995	WC	Tampere	GBR	6 28.11	
1962	WC	Lucerne	GER	6 54.6		1996	OG	Atlanta	GBR	6 20.09	
1963	EC	Copenhagen	ITA	6 53.3		1997	WC	Aiguebelette	FRA	6 27.69	
1964	EC	Amsterdam	NDL	6 42.6		1998	WC	Cologne	GER	6 22.32	
1964	OG	Tokyo	CAN	7 32.94		1999	WC	St Catharines	AUS	6 19.00	
1965	EC	Duisburg	DEN	7 29.3		2000	OG	Sydney	FRA	6 32.97	
1966	WC	Bled	RDA	6 53.96		2001	WC	Lucerne	GBR	6 27.57	
1967	EC	Vichy	USA	7 45.98		2002	WC	Seville	GBR	6 14.27	
1967	NAC	St Catharines	USA	7 21.5		2003	WC	Milano	AUS	6 19.31	
1968	OG	Mexico	RDA	7 26.56		2004	OG	Athens	AUS	6 30.76	
1969	EL	Klagenfurt	USA	7 11.73		2005	WC	Gifu	NZL	6 52.51	
1970	WC	St Catharines	RDA	6 57.81		2006	WC	Eton	AUS	6 18.00	
1971	EC	Copenhagen	RDA	6 43.40							

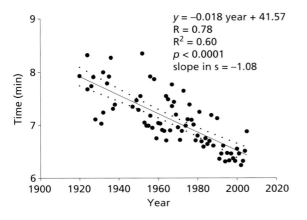

Fig. A.5 Men's pair.

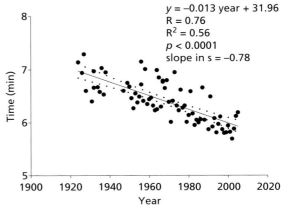

Fig. A.6 Men's four.

Table A.6 Winning results obtained in men's coxless four (M4–).

Year	Event	Place	Winner	Time (min s)	Comment	Year	Event	Place	Winner	Time (min s)	Comment
1900	OG	Paris	BEL	7 16.8	River	1953	EC	Copenhagen	DEN	6 33.2	
1904	OG	St Louis	USA	9 53.8	River	1954	EC	Amsterdam	ITA	6 22.8	
1908	OG	Henley	GBR	8 32.4	2414 m	1955	EC	Ghent	SUI	6 29.2	
1924	OG	Paris	GBR	7 08.6		1956	EC	Bled	ITA	6 42.9	
1925	EC	Prague	SUI	6 13.6	River	1956	OG	Melbourne	CAN	7 08.8	
1926	EC	Lucerne	SUI	6 56.2		1957	EC	Duisburg	GER	6 24.6	
1927	EC	Como	ITA	7 17.6		1958	EC	Poznan	GER	7 00.8	
1928	OG	Amsterdam	GBR	6 36.0		1959	EC	Macon	SUI	6 21.03	
1929	EC	Bydgoszcz	ITA	5 56.8	1750 m	1960	OG	Rome	USA	6 26.26	
1930	EC	Liege	ITA	5 53.4	River	1961	EC	Prague	ITA	6 28.29	
1931	EC	Paris	SUI	6 24		1962	WC	Lucerne	GER	6 19.24	
1932	EC	Belgrad	BON	6 39.8		1963	RC	Copenhagen	GER	6 13.88	
1932	OG	Los Angeles	GBR	6 58 2		1964	EC	Amsterdam	GER	6 15.10	
1933	EC	Budapest	DEN	6 04.6	2300 m	1964	OG	Tokyo	DEN	6 59.30	
1934	EC	Lucerne	GER	6 40.4		1965	EC	Duisburg	URS	6 50.99	
1935	EC	Berlin	SUI	6 34.9		1966	WC	Bled	RDA	6 18.41	
1936	OG	Berlin	GER	7 01.8		1967	EC	Vichy	RDA	6 47.50	
1937	EC	Amsterdam	GER	6 31.7		1967	NAC	St Catharines	RFA	6 46.41	
1938	EC	Milano	SUI	6 57.2		1968	OG	Mexico	RFA	6 39.18	
1947	EC	Lucerne	ITA	6 35.7		1969	EC	Klagenfurt	URS	6 47.90	
1948	OG	Henley	ITA	6 39.0	River	1970	WC	St Catharines	RDA	6 23.15	
1949	RC	Amsterdam	ITA	6 45.2		1971	EC	Copenhagen	RDA	6 00.72	
1950	EC	Milano	ITA	6 40.5		1972	OG	Munich	RDA	6 24.27	
1951	EC	Macon	BEL	6 27.8		1973	EC	Moscow	RDA	6 56.67	
1952	OG	Helsingfors	YOU	6 16.0		1974	WC	Lucerne	RDA	6 19.20	

(*Continued.*)

Table A.6 *Continued.*

Year	Event	Place	Winner	Time (min s)	Comment	Year	Event	Place	Winner	Time (min s)	Comment
1975	WC	Nottingham	RDA	6 13.81		1992	OG	Barcelona	AUS	5 55.04	
1976	OG	Montreal	RDA	6 37.42		1993	WC	Racice	FRA	6 04.54	
1977	WC	Amsterdam	RPA	6 16.73		1994	WC	Indianapolis	ITA	5 48.44	
1978	WC	L. Karapiro	URS	6 19.25		1995	WC	Tampere	ITA	5 58.28	
1979	WC	Bled	RDA	6 00.64		1996	OG	Atlanta	AUS	6 06.37	
1980	OG	Moscow	RDA	6 08.17		1997	WC	Aiguebelette	GBR	5 52.40	
1981	WC	Munich	URS	6 35.85		1998	WC	Cologne	GBR	5 48.06	
1982	WC	Lucerne	SUI	6 10.41		1999	WC	St Catharines	GBR	5 48.57	
1983	WC	Duisburg	RFA	5 57.02		2000	OG	Sydney	GBR	5 56.24	
1984	OG	Los Angeles	NZL	6 03.48		2001	WC	Lucerne	GBR	5 48.98	
1985	WC	Hazewinkel	RFA	6 00.19		2002	WC	Seville	GER	5 41.35	
1986	WC	Nottingham	USA	6 03.53		2003	WC	Milano	CAN	5 52.91	
1987	WC	Copenhagen	RDA	6 39.70		2004	OG	Athens	GBR	6 06.98	
1988	OG	Seoul	RDA	6 03.11		2005	WC	Gifu	GBR	6 11.59	
1990	WC	Tasmania	AUS	5 52.20		2006	WC	Eton	GBR	5 43.75	
1991	WC	Vienna	AUS	6 29.69							

Table A.7 Winning results in men's lightweight four (LM4–).

Year	Event	Place	Winner	Time (min s)	Year	Event	Place	Winner	Time (min s)
1974	WC	Lucerne	AUS	6 38.12	1991	WC	Vienna	GBR	5 57.60
1975	WC	Nottingham	FRA	6 47.31	1993	WC	Racice	USA	6 03.27
1976	WC	Villach	FRA	6 29.94	1994	WC	Indianapolis	DEN	5 53.77
1977	WC	Amsterdam	FRA	6 30.00	1995	WC	Tampere	ITA	6 16.46
1978	WC	Copenhagen	SUI	6 33.90	1996	OG	Atlanta	DEN	6 09.58
1979	WC	Bled	GBR	6 23.46	1997	WC	Aiguebelette	DEN	5 54.35
1980	WC	Hazewinkel	AUS	6 12.35	1998	WC	Cologne	DEN	6 01.53
1981	WC	Munich	AUS	6 22.32	1999	WC	St Catharines	DEN	6 45.63
1982	WC	Lucerne	ITA	6 17.79	2000	OG	Sydney	FRA	6 01.68
1983	WC	Duisburg	ESP	6 16.47	2001	WC	Lucerne	AUT	5 53.55
1984	WC	Montreal	ESP	6 09.39	2002	WC	Seville	DEN	5 47.21
1985	WC	Hazewinkel	RFA	6 12.44	2003	WC	Milano	DEN	6 10.46
1986	WC	Nottingham	ITA	6 18.26	2004	OG	Athens	DEN	6 01.39
1987	WC	Copenhagen	RFA	6 42.14	2005	WC	Gifu	FRA	5 47.91
1988	WC	Milan	ITA	6 09.48	2006	WC	Eton	CHN	5 49.43
1990	WC	Tasmania	GER	7 03.68					

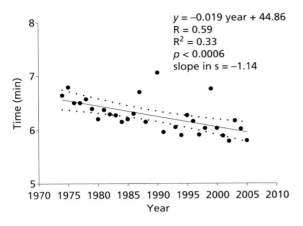

y = –0.019 year + 44.86
R = 0.59
R2 = 0.33
p < 0.0006
slope in s = –1.14
Time (min)
Year
8
7
6
5
1970
1975
1980
1985
1990
1995
2000
2005
2010

Fig. A.7 Lightweight men's four.

y = –0.01 year + 25.38
R = 0.69
R2 = 0.48
p < 0.0001
slope in s = –0.60
Time (min)
Year
8
7
6
5
1880
1900
1920
1940
1960
1980
2000
2020

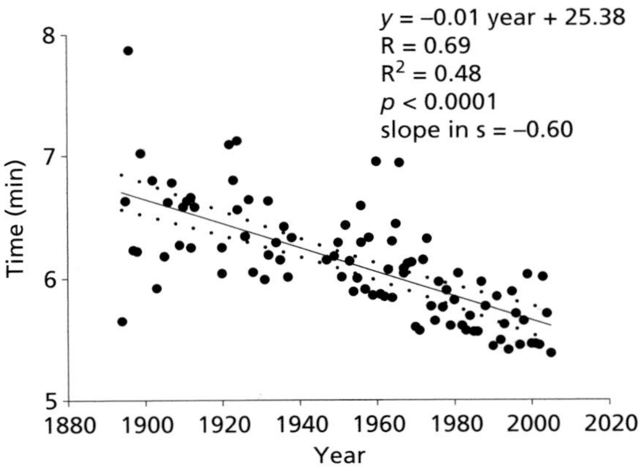

Fig. A.8 Men's coxed eight.

Table A.8 Winning results in men's eight (M8+).

Year	Event	Place	Winner	Time (min s)	Comment
1893	EC	Orta	FRA	10 14	3000 m
1894	EC	Macon	FRA	5 39	
1895	EC	Ostende	FRA	6 38	
1896	EC	Geneva	FRA	7 52	
1897	EC	Pallanza	BEL	6 14	
1898	EC	Torin	BEL	6 13	
1899	EC	Ostende	BEL	7 01	
1900	EC	Paris	BEL	5 24	1700 m
1900	OG	Paris	USA	6 09.8	River
1901	EC	Zürich	BEL	6 57	River
1902	EC	Strasbourg	BEL	6 48	
1903	EC	Venice	BEL	5 55	
1904	EC	Paris	BEL		
1904	OG	St Louis	USA	7 50.0	River
1905	EC	Ghent	FRA	6 11	
1906	EC	Pallanza	BEL	6 37	
1907	EC	Strasbourg	BEL	6 47	
1908	EC	Lucerne	BEL	6 45	River
1908	OG	Henley	GBR	7 56.0	2414 m
1909	EC	Juvisy	FRA	6 16	
1910	EC	Ostende	BEL	6 35	
1911	EC	Como	ITA	6 38	
1912	EC	Geneva	SUI	6 39.8	
1912	OG	Stockholm	GBR	6 15.0	
1913	EC	Ghent	GER	6 35	
1920	EC	Macon	SUI	6 15	
1920	OG	Antwerp	USA	6 02.6	
1921	EC	Amsterdam	SUI	6 40.6	1800 m
1922	EC	Barcelona	FRA	7 05.4	
1923	EC	Como	ITA	6 48	
1924	EC	Zürich	NDL	7 07	
1924	OG	Paris	USA	6 33.4	
1925	EC	Prague	SUI	5 41.8	River
1926	EC	Lucerne	NDL	6 20.6	
1927	EC	Como	ITA	6 38.4	
1928	OG	Amsterdam	USA	6 03.2	
1929	EC	Bydgoszcz	ITA	5 54.8	1750 m
1930	EC	Liege	USA	5 27.4	River
1931	EC	Paris	FRA	5 59 4	
1932	EC	Belgrad	YOU	6 11.4	
1932	OG	Los Angeles	USA	6 37.6	
1933	EC	Budapest	HON	5 44.2	2300 m
1934	EC	Lucerne	HON	6 17.4	
1935	EC	Berlin	HON	6 09.2	
1936	OG	Berlin	USA	6 25.4	
1937	EC	Amsterdam	ITA	6 00.5	
1938	EC	Milan	GER	6 19.9	
1947	EC	Lucerne	ITA	6 08.7	
1948	OG	Henley	USA	5 56.7	River
1949	EC	Amsterdam	ITA	6 11	

(*Continued.*)

Table A.8 *Continued.*

Year	Event	Place	Winner	Time (min s)	Comment	Year	Event	Place	Winner	Time (min s)	Comment
1950	RC	Milan	ITA	6 17.3		1977	WC	Amsterdam	RDA	5 45.36	
1951	EC	Macon	GBR	6 00.4		1978	WC	L. Karapiro	RDA	5 24.25	
1952	OG	Helsingfors	USA	6 25.9		1979	WC	Bled	RDA	5 36.41	
1953	EC	Copenhagen	URS	6 08.1		1980	OG	Moscow	RDA	5 49.05	
1954	EC	Amsterdam	URS	5 53.3		1981	WC	Munich	URS	6 02.30	
1955	EC	Ghent	HON	5 59.7		1982	WC	Lucerne	NZL	5 36.99	
1956	EC	Bled	TCH	6 17.5		1983	WC	Duisburg	NZL	5 34.39	
1956	OG	Melbourne	USA	6 35.2		1984	OG	Los Angeles	CAN	5 41.32	
1957	EC	Duisburg	ITA	5 54.3		1985	WC	Hazewinkel	URS	5 33.71	
1958	EC	Poznan	ITA	6 19.5		1986	WC	Nottingham	AUS	5 33.54	
1959	EC	Macon	GER	5 51.7		1987	WC	Copenhagen	USA	5 58.83	
1960	OG	Rome	GER	6 57.18		1988	OG	Seoul	RFA	5 46.05	
1961	EC	Prague	ITA	5 52.23		1990	WC	Tasmania	GER	5 26.62	
1962	WC	Lucerne	GER	5 50.83		1991	WC	Vienna	GER	5 50.98	
1963	EC	Copenhagen	GER	6 04.19		1992	OG	Barcelona	CAN	5 29.53	
1964	EC	Amsterdam	GER	5 50.60		1993	WC	Racice	GER	5 37.08	
1964	OG	Tokyo	USA	6 18.23		1994	WC	Indianapolis	USA	5 24.50	
1965	EC	Duisburg	GER	6 26.33		1995	WC	Tampere	GER	5 53.40	
1966	WC	Bled	RFA	6 56.28		1996	OG	Atlanta	NDL	5 42.74	
1967	EC	Vichy	RFA	6 04.89		1997	WC	Aiguebelette	USA	5 27.20	
1967	NAC	St Catharines	NZL	6 02.41		1998	WC	Cologne	USA	5 38.78	
1968	OG	Mexico	RFA	6 07.00		1999	WC	St Catharines	USA	6 01.58	
1969	EC	Klagenfurt	RDA	6 07.53		2000	OG	Sydney	ROM	5 27.48	
1970	WC	St Catharines	RDA	5 36.10		2001	WC	Lucerne	ROM	5 27.48	
1971	EC	Copenhagen	NZL	5 33.92		2002	WC	Seville	CAN	5 26.92	
1972	OG	Munich	NZL	6 08.94		2003	WC	Milano	CAN	6 00.44	
1973	EC	Moscow	RDA	6 19.02		2004	OG	Athens	USA	5 42.48	
1974	WC	Lucerne	USA	5 46.37		2005	WC	Gifu	USA	5 22.75	
1975	WC	Nottingham	RDA	5 39.01		2006	WC	Eton	GER	5 21.85	
1976	OG	Montreal	RDA	5 58.29							

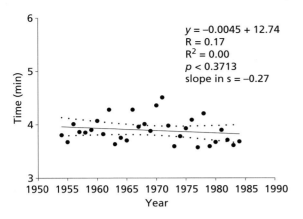

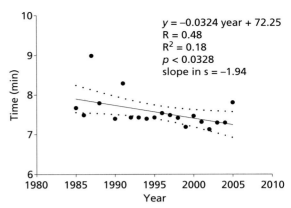

Fig. A.9 Women's single sculls (1000 m).

Fig. A.10 Women's single sculls (2000 m).

Table A.9 Winning results in women's single scull (W1x) over 1000 m.

Year	Event	Place	Winner	Time (min s)	Year	Event	Place	Winner	Time (min s)
1954	EC	Amsterdam	URS	3 48.1	1970	EC	Tata	RDA	4 21.62
1955	EC	Bukarest	URS	3 40.1	1971	EC	Copenhagen	RDA	4 30.75
1956	EC	Bled	RFA	4 00.6	1972	EC	Brandenburg	NDL	3 59.02
1957	EC	Duisburg	URS	3 51.7	1973	EC	Moscow	URS	3 59.02
1958	EC	Poznan	HaN	3 50.9	1974	WC	Lucerne	RDA	3 46.52
1959	EC	Macon	HaN	3 53.9	1975	WC	Nottingham	RDA	3 55.75
1960	RC	London	HON	4 04.40	1976	OG	Montreal	RDA	4 05.56
1961	EC	Prague	HaN	3 48.96	1977	WC	Amsterdam	RDA	3 34.31
1962	EC	Berlin	TCH	4 17.0	1978	WC	L. Karapiro	RDA	4 12.49
1963	EC	Moscow	URS	3 37.70	1979	WC	Bled	ROU	3 35.44
1964	EC	Amsterdam	URS	3 44.70	1980	OG	Moscow	ROD	3 40.69
1965	EC	Duisburg	URS	3 42.20	1981	WC	Munich	ROD	3 54.46
1966	EC	Amsterdam	URS	4 16.87	1982	WC	Lucerne	URS	3 42.83
1967	EC	Vichy	RDA	3 57.67	1983	WC	Duisburg	RDA	3 36.51
1968	EC	Berlin	RDA	4 00.79	1984	OG	Los Angeles	ROU	3 40.68
1969	EC	Klagenfurt	URS	3 53.01					

Table A.10 Winning results in women's single scull (W1x) over 2000 m.

Year	Event	Place	Winner	Time (min s)	Year	Event	Place	Winner	Time (min s)
1985	WC	Hazewinkel	RDA	7 40.37	1997	WC	Aiguebelette	BLR	7 29.30
1986	WC	Nottingham	RDA	7 29.60	1998	WC	Cologne	RUS	7 25.09
1987	WC	Copenhagen	BUL	8 59.26	1999	WC	St Catharines	BLR	7 11.68
1988	OG	Seoul	RDA	7 47.19	2000	OG	Sydney	BLR	7 28.14
1990	WC	Tasmania	GER	7 24.10	2001	WC	Lucerne	GER	7 19.25
1991	WC	Vienna	CAN	8 17.58	2002	WC	Seville	BUL	7 07.71
1992	OG	Barcelona	ROM	7 25.54	2003	WC	Milano	BUL	7 18.12
1993	WC	Racice	GER	7 26.00	2004	OG	Athens	GER	7 18.12
1994	WC	Indianapolis	DEN	7 23.96	2005	WC	Gifu	BLR	7 48.35
1995	WC	Tampere	SWE	7 26.00	2006	WC	Eton	BLR	7 11.02
1996	OG	Atlanta	BLR	7 32.21					

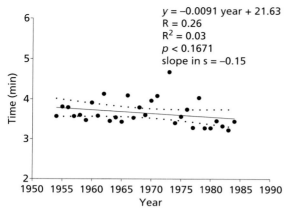

Fig. A.11 Women's double sculls (1000 m).

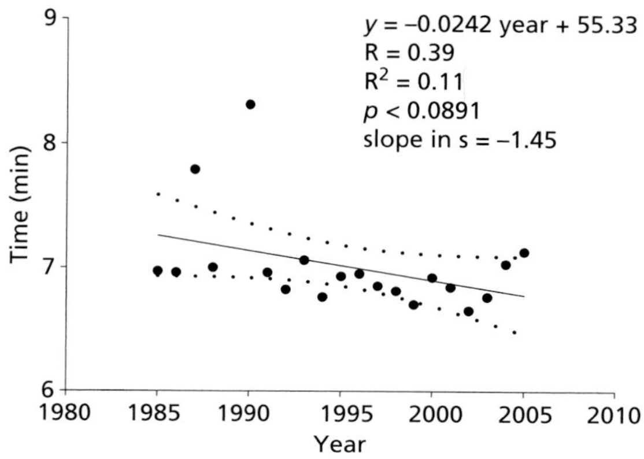

Fig. A.12 Women's double sculls (2000 m).

Table A.11 Winning results in women's double sculls (W2x) over 1000 m.

Year	Event	Place	Winner	Time min s	Year	Event	Place	Winner	Time min s
1954	EC	Amsterdam	URS	3 33.9	1970	EC	Tata	RDA	3 57.55
1955	EC	Bukarest	URS	3 48.4	1971	EC	Copenhagen	URS	4 04.55
1956	EC	Bled	TCH	3 17.5	1972	EC	Brandenburg	URS	
1957	EC	Duisburg	URS	3 34.0	1973	EC	Moscow	URS	3 40.05
1958	EC	Poznan	URS	3 36.0	1974	WC	Lucerne	URS	3 24.00
1959	EC	Macon	URS	3 28.0	1975	WC	Nottingham	URS	3 33.70
1960	EC	London	URS	3 54.75	1976	OG	Montreal	BUL	3 44.36
1961	EC	Prague	URS	3 34.92	1977	WC	Amsterdam	RDA	3 16.83
1962	EC	Berlin	URS	4 08.1	1978	WC	L. Karapiro	BUL	4 01.94
1963	EC	Moscow	URS	3 27.05	1979	WC	Bled	RDA	3 15.95
1964	EC	Amsterdam	URS	3 32.43	1980	OG	Moscow	URS	3 16.27
1965	EC	Duisburg	URS	3 25.56	1981	WC	Munich	URS	3 27.06
1966	EC	Amsterdam	RDA	4 05.21	1982	WC	Lucerne	URS	3 19.47
1967	EC	Vichy	URS	3 31.65	1983	WC	Duisburg	RDA	3 13.44
1968	EC	Berlin	RDA	3 47.13	1984	OG	Los Angeles	ROU	3 26.75
1969	EC	Klagenfurt	RDA	3 35.87					

Table A.12 Winning results in women's double sculls (W2x) over 2000 m.

Year	Event	Place	Winner	Time (min s)	Year	Event	Place	Winner	Time (min s)
1985	WC	Hazewinkel	RDA	6 58.80	1997	WC	Aiguebelette	GER	6 51.07
1986	WC	Nottingham	RDA	6 57.71	1998	WC	Cologne	GBR	6 48.85
1987	WC	Copenhagen	BUL	7 47.89	1999	WC	St Catharines	GER	6 41.98
1988	OG	Seoul	RDA	7 00.48	2000	OG	Sydney	GER	6 55.44
1990	WC	Tasmania	GER	8 18.63	2001	WC	Lucerne	GER	6 50.20
1991	WC	Vienna	CAN	6 57.42	2002	WC	Seville	NZL	6 38.78
1992	OG	Barcelona	GER	6 49.00	2003	WC	Milano	NZL	6 45.79
1993	WC	Racice	NZL	7 03.42	2004	OG	Athens	NZL	7 01.79
1994	WC	Indianapolis	NZL	6 45.30	2005	WC	Gifu	NZL	7 08.03
1995	WC	Tampere	CAN	6 55.76	2006	WC	Eton	AUS	6 47.67
1996	OG	Atlanta	CAN	6 56.84					

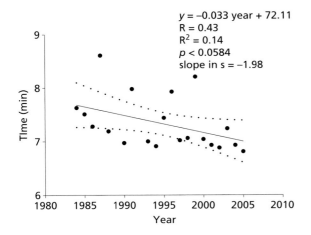

y = −0.033 year + 72.11
R = 0.43
R² = 0.14
p < 0.0584
slope in s = −1.98

Fig. A.13 Lightweight women's double sculls.

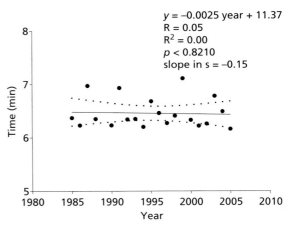

y = −0.0025 year + 11.37
R = 0.05
R² = 0.00
p < 0.8210
slope in s = −0.15

Fig. A.14 Women's quadruple sculls.

Table A.13 Winning results in women's light weight double sculls (LW2X).

Year	Event	Place	Winner	Time (min s)
1984	WC	Montreal	DEN	7 38.16
1985	WC	Hazewinkel	GBR	7 30.52
1986	WC	Nottingham	USA	7 17.13
1987	WC	Copenhagen	CAN	8 36.60
1988	WC	Milano	NDL	7 11.85
1990	WC	Tasmania	DEN	6 57.96
1991	WC	Vienna	GER	7 58.53
1993	WC	Racice	CAN	6 59.74
1994	WC	Indianapolis	CAN	6 54.85
1995	WC	Tampere	USA	7 26.45
1996	OG	Atlanta	USA	7 55.99
1997	WC	Aiguebelette	GER	7 00.93
1998	WC	Cologne	USA	7 03.73
1999	WC	St Catharines	ROM	8 12.67
2000	OG	Sydney	ROM	7 02.64
2001	WC	Lucerne	GER	6 55.55
2002	WC	Seville	AUS	6 52.84
2003	WC	Milano	GER	7 14.55
2004	OG	Athens	ROM	6 56.05
2005	WC	Gifu	GER	6 48.47
2006	WC	Eton	CHN	6 55.12

Table A.14 Winning results in women's quadruple scull over 2000 m.

Year	Event	Place	Winner	Time (min s)
1985	WC	Hazewinkel	RDA	6 22.47
1986	WC	Nottingham	RDA	6 13.91
1987	WC	Copenhagen	RDA	6 58.42
1988	OG	Seoul	RDA	6 21.06
1990	WC	Tasmania	GER	6 14.08
1991	WC	Vienna	GER	6 55.85
1992	OG	Barcelona	GER	6 20.18
1993	WC	Racice	CHN	6 21.07
1994	WC	Indianapolis	GER	6 11.73
1995	WC	Tampere	GER	6 40.80
1996	OG	Atlanta	GER	6 27.44
1997	WC	Aiguebelette	GER	6 16.15
1998	WC	Cologne	GER	6 24.38
1999	WC	St Catharines	GER	7 06.53
2000	OG	Sydney	GER	6 19.58
2001	WC	Lucerne	GER	6 12.95
2002	WC	Seville	GER	6 15.66
2003	WC	Milano	AUS	6 46.52
2004	OG	Athens	GER	6 29.29
2005	WC	Gifu	GBR	6 09.59
2006	WC	Eton	RUS	6 11.99

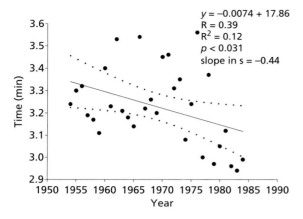

Fig. A.15 Women's coxed eight (1000 m).

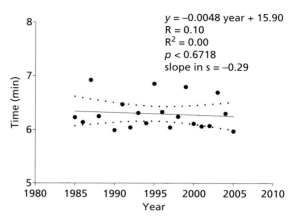

Fig. A.16 Women's coxed eight (2000 m).

Table A.15 Winning results in women eight (W8+) over 1000 m.

Year	Event	Place	Winner	Time (min s)
1954	EC	Amsterdam	URS	3 14.5
1955	EC	Bukarest	URS	3 17.8
1956	EC	Bled	URS	3 19.4
1957	EC	Duisburg	URS	3 11.4
1958	EC	Poznan	URS	3 10.3
1959	EC	Macon	URS	3 06.3
1960	EC	London	URS	3 23.70
1961	EC	Prague	URS	3 13.59
1962	EC	Berlin	URS	3 32.00
1963	EC	Moscow	URS	3 12.75
1964	EC	Amsterdam	RDA	3 10.63
1965	EC	Duisburg	URS	3 08.13
1966	EC	Amsterdam	RDA	3 32.41
1967	EC	Vichy	URS	3 13.20
1968	EC	Berlin	RDA	3 15.62
1969	EC	Klagenfurt	RDA	3 11.92
1970	EC	Tata	RDA	3 27.05
1971	EC	Copenhagen	URS	3 27.78
1972	EC	Brandenburg	URS	3 18.53
1973	EC	Moscow	URS	3 21.12
1974	WC	Lucerne	RDA	3 04.82
1975	WC	Nottingham	RDA	3 14.53
1976	OG	Montreal	RDA	3 33.32
1977	WC	Amsterdam	RDA	3 00.23
1978	WC	L. Karapiro	URS	3 22.00
1979	WC	Bled	URS	2 58.09
1980	OG	Moscow	RDA	3 03.32
1981	WC	Munich	URS	3 07.58
1982	WC	Lucerne	URS	2 57.97
1983	WC	Duisburg	URS	2 56.22
1984	OG	Los Angeles	USA	2 59.80

Table A.16 Winning results in women eight (W8+) over 2000 m.

Year	Event	Place	Winner	Time (min s)
1985	WC	Hazewinkel	URS	6 14.00
1986	WC	Nottingham	URS	6 08.76
1987	WC	Copenhagen	ROU	6 55.61
1988	OG	Seoul	RDA	6 15.17
1990	WC	Tasmania	ROM	5 59.26
1991	WC	Vienna	CAN	6 28.20
1992	OG	Barcelona	CAN	6 02.62
1993	WC	Racice	ROM	6 18.88
1994	WC	Indianapolis	GER	6 07.42
1995	WC	Tampere	USA	6 50.73
1996	OG	Atlanta	ROM	6 19.73
1997	WC	Aiguebelette	ROM	6 02.40
1998	WC	Cologne	ROM	6 14.62
1999	WC	St Catharines	ROM	6 47.66
2000	OG	Sydney	ROM	6 06.44
2001	WC	Lucerne	AUS	6 03.66
2002	WC	Seville	USA	6 04.25
2003	WC	Milano	GER	6 41.23
2004	OG	Athens	ROM	6 17.70
2005	WC	Gifu	AUS	5 58.10
2006	WC	Eton	USA	5 55.50

Index

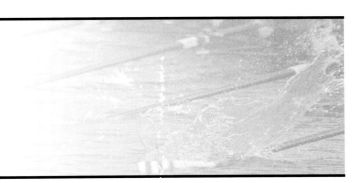

sculling
   blade area   25–6
   injuries   126–7
   professional   10
   span   *23*, 24
seat(s)
   coxswain's   125
   distance of travel   *23*, 24
   height   *23*, 24
   sliding   12, 35
seat racing   97–9
seating arrangement   *146*
selection of rowers   97–9, 152
self-belief   79
self-confidence   79
self-statements, positive   82
semi-professional status   20
shoulder, wheelchair users   143
showering   129
sitting height   35
six-minute all-out effort   42
skeletal muscle
   blood flow   59
   characteristics   39–41
   function/structure   121–2
skin
   heat exchange   134–5
   infections   133
   temperature   134
skinfold thickness measurement
      104, *106*
sleeping tablets   131
slide angle   *23*, 24
sliding riggers   11–12
sloeproeien   8
slow twitch muscle fibers   39–40,
      53
   central fatigue   61, 64
snacks
   carbohydrate-rich   **105**, 110,
      111
   competition venues   112
   nutrient-rich   104
   pre-/post-race   112
   protein   104
sodium chloride loss   135
sodium cromoglycate   132
Spain   3
span, sculling   *23*, 24
specialization in training   87
SpeedCoach™   34
spinal cord injuries   141–4
   doping of rowers   138–9
   exercise response   141–3
spine curvature   115–16
spondylolysis   127
sports medicine   124–39
   anti-doping   136–9
   health assessment   132–3
   injuries   126–9
   safety   124–6
   water-borne diseases   129–30
sprint, effectiveness   90

stadia   152
Staphylococcus aureus skin
      infections   133
Starling's law of the heart   54
staying in the moment   78
steering   126, 145–50
   tips   148–50
stimulants   136, 137
strength   90–2
   development phases   93
   endurance   92
   general   91
   maximum   90
   relative   90–1
   specific   91
strength training   92–5
   accumulation   93–4
   intensification   94
   methods   92–3
   microcycles   95
   periodization   93–4
   planning   93–4
   preparatory cycle   93–4
   program   87
   racing cycle   94
   transition cycle   94
stress   75, 80
   physiologic in competitive
      events   68
stressors, exposure to   66
stretcher angle   *23*, 24
stretcher force   28
stretcher position   *23*, 24
stretching programs   127, 133
stroke
   assessment   97, *98*
   rate   27
stroke cycle
   key events   **31**
   microphases   28, *29*, *30*, **31**
   timing   28
stroke rowers, muscle fibers   40
stroke volume   57
   demand   55
   exercising paraplegics   142–3
StrokeCoach   34
style of rowing   13, 16–17, 30–3
   changes   152
substitutions of rowers   132
succinate dehydrogenase   40
supercompensation   85, *86*
supplements
   history   133
   liquid meal   **113**
   use   112–13
surf boat rowing   9–10
sweating   109, 135
sweep rowers
   body build   36
   injuries   126–7
   low back pain   127
swimming certificates   124
sympathetic activity   59

sympatho-adrenergic system   71
syncope, vasovagal   54

T cells   68–9
tachycardia, exercise   57
talent identification   153
tanks, rowing   13, *16*, 153
technique of rowing   30–4
   effective   28
   improvement   153
telemetric oxygen uptake monitor
      42
temperature, body   133, 134
   brain   64
   elevation   52
   skin   134
temperature, environmental   133
   mean radiant   134
   training effects   134–5
   water   126, 136
   wet bulb globe   134
tenosynovitis, wrist   126–7, 128
terbutaline   132, 138
testosterone   71
Thames watermen races   3
Therapeutic Use Exemptions
      (TUEs)   *138*
   see also Abbreviated Therapeutic
      Use Exemption (ATUE)
thought stopping techniques   80
thoughts, positive/negative   78–81
tidal volume   48
time regulations   126
Tomkins, James   7
total lung capacity   48
traffic regulations   124–5, 126
traineras   3
training   85–95, 152
   active participation   88–9
   aerobic capacity   89–90
   camps   153
   complexity   87
   deterioration   66
   energy requirements   108
   enhanced   152
   failure of adaptation   66, 67, 73
   flexibility   86
   frequency   85
   fuelling   109–11
   hydration   109
   immediate effects   85
   individualization   87–8
   intensity   67–8, 85, **91**
   load in FES rowing   143–4
   methods   85
   micronutrient requirements
      108–9
   multilateral development   87
   nutrient-rich snacks   104
   nutrition guidelines   108–11
   opportunities   152–3
   periodization   88
   program   73